GLUTEN, SUGAR, STARCH:

HOW TO FREE YOURSELF FROM THE FOOD ADDICTIONS THAT ARE RAVAGING YOUR HEALTH AND KEEPING YOU FAT

A PALEO APPROACH

By Eric Morrison

LEGAL DISCLAIMER

The information contained in this book is not intended to be a replacement for professional medical advice. It is not meant to diagnose or treat any medical condition. It is strongly urged that you consult with your primary health care provider or naturopath to diagnose any medical condition and to discuss the ideas contained in this book before attempting to make any dietary changes. Should you and your care provider decide that it would be permissible for you to apply the ideas contained in this book, you do so at your own risk and take full responsibility for your actions.

The author is not liable for any damages or injury resulting from any action by a person reading or following the information in this book.

Table of Contents

INTRODUCTION 7

SECTION I: PROCESSED AND OTHER HARMFUL FOODS – BREAKING THE
ADDICTION 22

Part I: Your Addiction to Gluten 26

Part II: Your Addiction to Sugar 37

Part III: Your Addiction to Starches 50

Part IV: Other Toxic Consumable Goods 60

Part V: A Word About Alcohol 70

SECTION II: NATURAL FOODS – THE GENESIS OF YOUR APPROVED LIST 75

Part I: Nuts and Seeds 87

Part II: Fruits 90

Part III: Vegetables 93

Part IV: Nightshades 95

Part V: Dairy (And Fermented Dairy)...97

Part VI: Fermented Foods..100

Part VII: Fish and Seafood..103

Part VIII: Poultry and Avian Game Meats 107

Part IX: Pork and Wild Boar 110

Part X: Red Meats—Beef, Bison/Buffalo, Veal, Venison, Lamb and Elk 115

Part XI: Water 118

Appendix I: Now That You're Paleo..122

Appendix II: Can I Be Paleo and Vegan? 127

Appendix III: Converting A Family Over to Paleo-Style Eating....................132

Appendix IV: The Timing of Meals and Fasting 134

Appendix V: The Author's Personal Approved List—A Template for Creating
Your Own...138

INTRODUCTION

This is a book about paleo eating. If you haven't heard of the paleo diet by now you'd be a rarity in this media-saturated modern world of ours. The trend is hot. No doubt about it. And it's hot because it works. And people are reporting astounding results when switching to a paleo form of eating. They report both incredible positive changes in their overall health and unprecedented weight loss.

Paleo eating is a revelation in this modern age of processed and convenience foods. The concept of paleo is boiled down to this. Eat like our ancestors (from the Paleolithic era of humanity), not like those of us who can nowadays go to the store and fuel up on Twinkies and Coca-Cola whenever we want. In other words, *eat like a caveman.* If you lived on Earth a few thousand years ago instead of in our present day, the thinking goes that if you couldn't go out and dig it up, pick it from a bush or tree, fish for it or otherwise kill it then you wouldn't eat it. There was no refining or processing involved. The technology to do so just wasn't available. So the basis for this eating plan isn't so much what a caveman would eat but rather what he *couldn't eat.* This is really the proper consideration when attempting to identify whether or not a food choice can be called paleo. Cooking over fire was likely to have been utilized in the preparation of many meals to make them more tender or tasty but that would be about all of the toying a caveman could have done with their food. However, this entire ideology excludes a tremendous amount of things that we modern humans have become accustomed to and fond of in our normal diets these days, especially grains and added sugar. Actually, the effort to avoid just these two staples alone represents a gigantic amount of things that need to be excluded directly from our grocery store shelves. One or both of these substances are found in nearly *everything* that is categorized as processed food.

The paleo way isn't really a diet, necessarily. It's considered more of a *lifestyle transformation.* Think of it as a transitioning from previous staple foods and a way of eating to a whole new set of previously unimagined rules of subsistence. Once adopted, the eating style is intended to be permanent. And while it is not necessarily a weight loss model, absurd amounts of weight loss will absolutely result when the plan is followed properly. In fact, if the eating style does become adopted long-term as it is intended, it can be expected that the person living that way will revert to their natural body weight over time. The natural body weight of a person will vary depending on their gender, age, height and other factors. Since fit women naturally carry more body fat than fit men, women that have fully acclimated to the paleo eating style can expect to slim down to the 21-24% body fat range while men are more likely to reach the 14-17% body fat range once they have done the same. Further, they can expect to see all signs of visible fat (along with visceral fat) eventually disappear. The time frame for these effects to become fully realized, obviously, would be dictated by the amount of body fat the person has accumulated on their body prior to executing the lifestyle switch. Logically, if *permanent* weight loss is your motivation for going paleo, then a *permanent* switch over to the eating style must be made. But, paleo living is so much more a recipe for vastly improved health than anything else. Strict paleo wisdom blames our common modern killers (obesity, diabetes, heart disease and even cancer) on the food we eat. As the logic goes, cleaning that aspect of our lives up will reverse such conditions.

Basic paleo thinking states the following:

1.) Everything that we've been told is good for us to consume within the past century mostly isn't. And, 2.) modern processed and convenience foods must be eliminated as these foods are destroying the health of people across the globe and are most responsible for the global obesity epidemic.

On a paleo plan, these processed foods are replaced mostly by natural foods in their pristine untouched state. Only minimal processing such as seasoning, the blending of ingredients and/or the use of approved cooking methods is usually permitted.

While the whole idea appears reasonable enough on the surface, switching over to a paleo-inspired style of eating is not for the faint of heart.

That is where this book finds its niche. There are enough books out now on the "what" and "why" of paleo eating. This isn't another of those. This book instead seeks to solve the major problem that exists with *transitioning* to a paleo way of eating. We'll call it the first book on "how" to do it right. No book I've read yet adequately addresses this issue.

Why is transitioning over to a paleo eating style so difficult?

Paleo programs mean well and definitely do deliver for those who successfully make the transition to the paleo lifestyle. But, let's for a moment consider what it means to "successfully make the transition" for the average modern consumer. This is likely someone who has subsisted, perhaps for their entire life, on a low-fat, high-carb diet (because that is what has been dogmatically reported as being the "healthy" diet for the past seven decades). We are talking about someone who eats processed, refined foods for every meal, every take out order, every snack between meals and who probably washes every sitting down with sodas (diet, or not), energy drinks or sweetened teas and juices. This could also be someone who has been told they are eating healthy because most of their choices are low in, that most insidious of historic health saboteurs, saturated fat.

Now tell them what they can't eat anymore... According to paleo thinking, *everything* that this person lives on has to go.

Yikes! Sell that one, P.T. Barnum.

The gap between what common paleo wisdom espouses and what modern consumers call a meal is surely vast. Paleo eating is essentially the equivalent of the strictest *elimination diet* imaginable. It eliminates pretty much everything the average modern consumer has grown to love.

So how do you make a paleo book that would appeal to (and succeed for) someone who says they are open to making a "lifestyle change" as long as they don't have to give up Ding-Dongs? Or who can't see themselves giving up their morning whole wheat toast (that they proudly slather with fat-free margarine) because it is made from healthy whole grains? Or who says they can *eat right* all day long but when 8 pm rolls around each night and they start thinking about ice cream they cannot seem to resist the temptation to indulge in it?

Fair questions, to be sure. And they are *tough* questions on top of that. The answer is to take an almost *anti-paleo* angle at first. Paleo adaptation is packaged as an all-at-once, take no prisoners type of all-or-nothing approach to making an eating change. Take a close look at paleo books written to date. None of them really present an easy assimilation into the lifestyle. Sugar is bad. Beans are bad. Grains are bad. Deal with it. Drop it all now and make the switch or you will stay fat, sick and unhappy.

Good luck with that...

This strategy simply won't work where we are at as a society today and we have the psychology of the human being to thank for it. Take a strict paleo approach and tell someone as described above that it is time to get rid of their comfort foods and make a switch to a more obedient, conscientious way of thinking about food and you will surely produce someone with "dug-in" heels and a devout resistance to anything you're trying to sell. Guaranteed.

We love our comfort foods. They fulfill so much more for our bodies (and for our psyche) than just providing us with nutrients. They are powerful. Powerful, and misunderstood. But, we'll get to that in a minute. For most, they are the reason the heels get dug in in the first place. It feels as though, as much as we know we should give these foods up, we can't ever see ourselves living without certain ones.

Compounding the problem with these comfort foods even further is the one thing we haven't addressed yet, which is the prime focus of this book itself. It is a problem so under-appreciated that it is nearly non-existent as a news item but still is a very real condition in the world of nutrition and self-healing. We may very well be *addicted* to our favorite foods.

I mean this in a very literal sense. I am talking about food addictions and the process of becoming *addicted*. Addicted, as in the same way a drug addict or alcohol abuser becomes hooked on the chemicals that alter their own brain's chemistry to produce an effect. This is the same effect that they rely on the "drug" that they covet to produce for them again and again.

This is no joke. Plenty of research has been done to confirm the fact that receptors in the human brain respond very similarly when fed both substances—illicit drugs (or alcohol) or processed, refined foods (primarily grain flours and sugars). These receptors also react the same way (by creating withdrawal symptoms) when repeated long-term use of either of these substances suddenly ceases. There are treatment facilities (or rehab centers, if you will) for food addictions springing up all across the country. Don't believe me? Consult the search engines. It is a very real problem.

The symptoms of food *withdrawal* are not at all unlike those that drug or alcohol withdrawal can produce—dizziness, insomnia, diarrhea, stomach pain, headaches, etc. Not to mention, unbearable cravings for the substance, or in this case, the food ingredient that one is trying to recover from.

OK, so now, with all of this also in mind, let's look again at the task of converting an average consumer over to a paleo eating plan.

Talk about an assault on someone's personal level of comfort. As far as the degree to which a switch to a particular eating plan will threaten the comfort level of an individual enjoying the typical modern diet, a transition to paleo-style eating has got to rank among the highest. No question about it.

On top of the sudden loss of all of their favorite foods, which is probably already enough deterrent for most, let's add in the fact that the subject in question will also most assuredly experience some degree of withdrawal symptoms from the removal of the foods to which they are addicted. These symptoms are usually not very pleasant and can make the subject long so deeply for the missing substances, with their lure of alleviating the symptoms once they appear, that they alone are usually enough to cause them to cave in.

Don't get me wrong. Paleo-style eating, once one becomes adapted to it, is a fantastic and wonderful way to live. Its merits continue to be proven to me consistently, each and every day and I have eaten this way faithfully for over two years now. The change for me has cured poor circulation, erectile dysfunction, high blood pressure, back and body aches and has me parked at 15% body fat (down from a peak of 30%). And the *energy*! The boundless energy that now fuels my days has been worth making the change all by itself. The science is out there. The headlines aren't lying. Paleo eating is superior to the way most modern humans are eating in this fast-paced modern world. Most people are coming around to this idea. But jumping right into a paleo type of eating plan for someone who eats the way the person described above does would be something like standing at the base of Mt. Everest and preparing for the first step up the sucker. It truly will seem like it can't be done for this person (who, by the way, turns out to describe a very large percentage of the world's population). For them, the benefits of paleo might never be experienced and the plan will forever be just another crazy diet they couldn't stick to because it was too ridiculous in the first place. This needs to change.

Well, I have good news. It can be done. You can make a complete transition over to a paleo lifestyle. And somewhat painlessly, in contrast to the way described above. This book is the way to make it all happen.

I argue in this book that paleo eating is the only way to stay away from the doctor's office in this age of an ever-increasing worldwide health crisis. However, my contention is that sedentary modern human beings eating a traditionally recommended diet are not equipped with the ability to make an overnight shift to paleo. It would take an extraordinary person with incredible resolve and willpower to break from a modern processed diet and instantaneously move to a purely paleo plan. You might be that person but, more likely, this monumental task will be better accomplished over time. Gradually. And it will require a strategy that includes a well-written, easy to follow procedure for doing so. This book is that plan.

So just how did we, as a species, get to where we are today with our obesity reaching epidemic proportions and our collective health in crisis?

As a culture, we have been bombarded with a huge host of misinformation within the last century. The USDA's "Food Pyramid," with its advice to eat low-fat and adhere to a very rigid regimen of cramming grain-based after grain-based snack or meal six to eleven times a day into our pie-holes, should be difficult for just about anyone to stick to. After all, who eats eleven times a day? Even if you are trying to follow their updated and slightly more relaxed "My Plate" recommendations, the low-fat, high-carbohydrate eating plan is still foisted as the ideal human diet. But, I think for some of us this would seem rather indulgent. Are "reduced-fat" Oreo's just as acceptable as a snack choice from a nutritional standpoint as a side of steamed broccoli? I think I'll pass on hearing about the justification for that logic. Yet, these are the sort of recommendations for "healthy" food choices being offered by our officials in charge of this aspect of our lives. Do we really need officials appointed to this part of our normal existence? Can't we figure this part out for ourselves? If we eat it and we don't feel so good a few hours later, shouldn't we question whether or not that is the right food for us to return to meal after meal?

This book will absolutely fly right in the face of just about everything we have been told by nutrition "experts" and even our own medical professionals for the past seven decades all the way back to the "basic seven" of 1946.

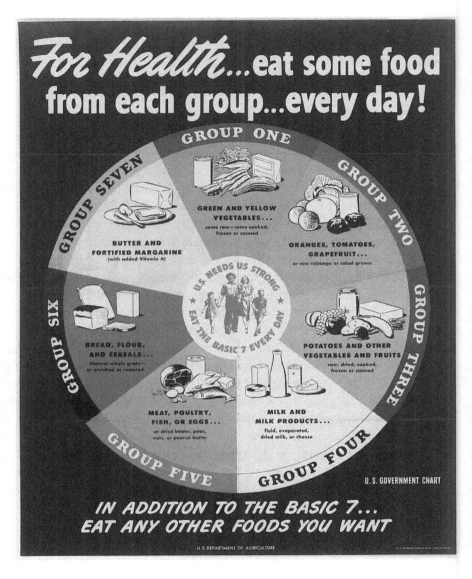

I especially love the above encouragement to "eat any other foods you want" in addition to these seven foods listed. What kind of recommendation for a healthy diet is this anyway? It sounds a lot like the recommendation is "well, here's seven foods we think might be healthy, but, you know what? The hell with it. Just eat whatever you want to."

I will ask that you put this 70 or so years of conditioning aside only long enough to review what I will present. Could the experts have been wrong all this time? My opinion is absolutely, yes. Was the bad advice given motivated with an intentional purpose in mind or was it just a product of poor science? For all you conspiracy theorists, that debate is for another day. But, you will likely come around to my way of thinking about the (lack of) efficacy of these programs before you finish this book. Keep an open mind.

As I previously mentioned, I have been adhering to a paleo-inspired eating style for over two years now. I say "paleo-inspired" because that is the way of eating which most closely resembles the way I actually eat now. There are lots of subdivisions of what some may call "paleo," however. It can become almost comical at times seeing the ways that certain proponents of the diet arrive at just what it is that "a caveman would eat." I see *strict paleo* advocates harping on the details of their diet, the "strictest" aspect of which includes the abandonment of dairy products (milk, yogurt, cheese, etc.) yet they cook all their paleo meals in ghee (clarified butter) because it holds up to high-heat cooking without the risk of dangerous oxidization. Another example... No matter how strict a paleo eater might be, it seems almost universally acceptable within the paleo community to use coconut oil in everything. But, I have a hard time envisioning a caveman making oil from coconuts. I think it also would have been pretty difficult for early Paleolithic man living in what is now the mid-western section of the United States to even find a coconut.

So while, I poke a little fun at the movement, I am also very grateful for each and every one of the very dedicated proponents of the paleo lifestyle, for without them I would not be as invigorated and fired-up about eating the right things for my body as I am today. But, I am trying to not *think* paleo anymore. It isn't something I consciously labor over in my food choices these days. I don't really stop to consider whether a caveman would have had a French press or not. Is it going to stop me from sucking down my morning coffee? Not hardly. However, there is no doubt that, no matter what I pick to eat, it will be accepted by at least one of the generally-recognized categories of paleo eating.

This is because I have developed my very own list of foods that I can eat—foods that make me feel great and perform at peak levels. I also have a list of foods that don't work for me. These are foods that can be addictive, destructive or which have proven to make me feel lousy after I eat them.

These are the *excluded* and *approved* food lists which govern my food choices these days. They aren't really written down any more but rather reside in my head as a sort of paleo common sense. But at first they were written down (my own personal approved list is included for reference as an appendix in the back of this book). They were hatched from a paleo platform and became somewhat modified to suit my personal food tolerances.

I will teach you how to create your own such lists in this book. We will start you out with an excluded list which will be developed from the beginning section of this book on breaking addictions. Then you will create your approved list in the following section. Once you have this second list, you won't have a great need to hang on to your excluded list. If it doesn't appear on the approved list, it isn't to be eaten. Eventually, your approved list will become memorized (as mine is) and won't need to be retained as a physical list any longer either.

Your lists should be different from mine. The individual physiology of every human being seems to differ, one from another, in what each is able to tolerate in the foods they consume.

I am not trying to change the paleo world with some bright new offering on how things should be done. Then again, maybe I am. But, my foremost goal is to present a thoughtful way to assist those who can't see themselves ever being able to make the extreme transition to a paleo way of eating from their ineffective, yet familiar low-fat, high-carb way of doing things. I am trying to lessen the incidence of *paleo fall-out*. We don't hear about the failure rate for the paleo way of eating. I'm not saying the eating style is a failure, but rather that the rates of latching on to it as a newbie and successfully turning it into a permanent way of life might be lower than we think. We don't know. All we see on the blogs are story after story of how fantastic eating that way is. And it is. But, do we really think that switching over to this way of life is easy and people all over the world are having no trouble at all with it and everybody converts? Without any figures to back me up, I am going to say... uh, no.

Deprivation and fear of hunger are very real concerns for someone considering a paleo-type plan. I made the switch a little more naturally than I imagine most would. But, I was coming from changes I had already made in my life starting with a low-carb, moderate-protein program, adding in gluten-free eating on top of it and then transitioning into a paleo form of eating. And even though paleo eating isn't really concerned with counting calories or carbs nor does it utilize any other form of food rationing, it was still *very difficult*. It got me to thinking about a better way...

So, let me comfort you somewhat by telling you that there is no enormous radical change needing to be made right away to get to paleo world using my strategies.

Does that help a little bit?

I want to get you there and the sooner the better. You will need to adjust to the changes you will be making to your way of eating one by one, but you are still going to get there when you get there. You won't be dieting; you will *be rehabilitating*. Rehabilitating from the crippling substances in your food that have been robbing you of your health, training your mind and destroying your body image. It is very possible that this will be a very long and difficult process. Taking the example of the lifelong low-fat, high-carb eater, they are likely addicted to *many more than just one substance* in their food that produces effects for them. The road to paleo will be a lot longer for them. But it shouldn't be any more difficult than it would be for anyone else, just longer. That is the beauty of what I have discovered and offer in this book.

Rehab isn't fun. It isn't fun for the drug addict and it isn't fun for those with a similar addiction to the foods they eat. But, I promise to those who persist through the rehab process, the grass is really greener on the other side. As you free yourself from the grip of one substance that is harmful and doesn't want to let go, you tend to replace it with many more that are loaded with nutrients that the human body thrives on and that do not have any addictive hold over you. You eat them enthusiastically because you've discovered that you love them, not because you get a headache when it's been too long since the last time you had a serving of them.

Eventually, as I stated earlier, you will develop a personal list of your own of excluded foods that will be populated with all of your very own paleo no-no's (irrespective of the version of paleo you began with). And then the list will be increased, if needed, by anything else that might not agree with you.

That will be the main context of this book going forward, "does it work for you?"

No issues? Then it gets forwarded to your approved list as a permanent staple. If not, then it disappears from your own personal list of what works, forever.

This isn't a diet and, as you may be able to tell, it won't be a one-size-fits-all eating plan either. You will be cleaning your pantry and refrigerator of all the foods you are addicted to and that have been causing you so much harm without you even realizing it. I am excited to tell you that you don't even know how good you are going to feel once you have your approved list completed and are able to eat any amount of any food on the list without needing to count calories or carbohydrates or fat or anything else you might feel compelled to count. Eat them all without guilt. For the rest of your life, these will be your foods—the foods *your* body is meant to run on.

The easiest way for a food to land on the approved list is if it meets the following criteria:

"I feel fantastic when I eat this food"

or,

"I feel no change when I eat this food"

Anything short of these has got to go.

Bloating and gastric cramping are not normal conditions for the human body to experience. Extreme peaks and lows in energy levels aren't normal either and represent irregularities in insulin production. These are but two examples of hundreds of negative conditions within the body that are normally always brought about by consuming the wrong foods for a person's genetic makeup.

Every person's genetic makeup is different and each one's tolerance to certain food types will vary but the process to figure out what works for you (and also what doesn't) is not going to require expensive blood panel testing or other medical testing procedures. You are simply going to become a guinea pig for your own health. No medical test in the world will be able to give you a better indication of whether or not a certain type of food is the culprit for a certain one of your symptoms than your very own body can. Don't wait for the lab results. Ask yourself "how do I feel after I eat it?"

This is not designed as a weight loss book whatsoever. And I share this because the success of getting to where you want to go depends on following the rules for doing so as set forth in this book and not double-checking progress with a scale. Weight loss beyond your wildest dreams will start to happen as you progress through the stages of arriving at a paleo form of eating. It is a side effect of eating what your body is intended by nature to be fueled on. But, you should not be in a hurry to lose weight.

Successful rehabilitation depends on replacement – one destructive habit for one or more healthy ones. It doesn't happen overnight and neither should fully adapting to a paleo way of eating. It could take a year or so to say that you are truly eating paleo. And that is OK because, along the way, there will come moments when you can look back at your previous menu for a normal day for your formerly addicted self and be overcome with pride at how much you've accomplished in cleaning up your body and in working to break every single one of your food addictions.

The deprivation and fear of hunger that I spoke about earlier should not show up as concerns for you while using this program of conversion to paleo. The only thing that you will find that you will become deprived of along the way will be the toxic and fattening foods that trick your mind into craving more and more. Once your brain gets used to the replacement for each of these foods, you will not miss them, I promise. But that is once you break the addiction. Because those kinds of food will not give up without a fight. Of this you can be sure. Your brain will no doubt whisper in your ear and tell you that you are being deprived but, from a nutritional standpoint, no lie could be greater. As for hunger, it should not be a problem either because you are training your system to adjust to a new way of eating at an extremely reasonable rate. Your stomach may not even catch on, to be honest.

Have patience and follow along with the guidelines in this book *at your own pace*. Pay no attention to the urgings of your friends who are already doing their 100% paleo diets. They will be very poor resources for you as you work through this book. They have a completely different mindset than you do right now. It won't mesh very well with yours at this point. But, you'll get there. Just remember, every person's genetic makeup is different, so therefore every person's acclimation to the stages of transition on this journey to what will eventually be considered true paleo eating 100% of the time will happen at different rates. You will be doing the exact opposite of what other paleo plans would prescribe which is dump everything you love right now and dive right in to only eating foods you haven't eaten since the last time your mother forced you to stay at the table until they were gone. Not a very calculated recipe for success, I feel. You, on the other hand, will be breaking addictions one by one to eventually arrive at a very profound goal. This is a dietary goal that if you had to switch to overnight would not interest you in the slightest.

One final note. This book will not be written in an exhaustively scientific or technical manner. If that's your thing, I would steer you to books by Gary Taubes, Dr. Loren Cordain or Dr. William Davis for your validation of the science behind paleo. Mine, on the other hand, is more of a *how to get there* book rather than a *why it will work* book.

My approach is simple.

I think a deep green leafy salad beats a Ding Dong any day of the week. If you agree with me but still find yourself consistently making the wrong choice when the two are sitting in front of you, then this is the book for you.

Let's get busy. There's much work to be done.

SECTION I: PROCESSED AND OTHER HARMFUL FOODS – BREAKING THE ADDICTION

Voltaire is credited with exclaiming that "common sense is not so common." This pretty much hits the current obesity epidemic/health crisis right on its proverbial head. You will start to see as you progress along in this section how your own common sense in making healthy food choices has been adversely influenced by both "expert" recommendations as well as the power of your own addicted brain to obscure the facts.

This section on addictions will zero in on the foods in a typical American diet that are likely to be causing an addictive effect in their consumers without them even knowing it.

"Being hungry" for Doritos does not imply that one's body is deeply desiring the nutritive value of the elements found in Doritos snack chips. That is very likely not the case at all. Yet, I have heard this argument before.

"Well, there must be something in Doritos that my body needs or I wouldn't be wanting some right now."

I beg to differ.

If you are a regular consumer of Doritos (and perhaps you are), your body stays engaged in a very demanding battle to constantly recover from the effects of the toxic agents contained within this unassuming snack. In truth, the "hunger" you feel is a craving produced by your brain for the substance that produces an effect of which your brain has become conditioned to receive. There are actually *several* compounds within a Dorito chip which could be the culprit, not just one. And this is the case with most processed food. *"We need more of that"* your brain-washed brain has decided. In fact, the "hunger" your brain can produce in an addicted state can be so incredibly powerful that it may leave you writhing in pain and convinced you will die if you don't get something in your belly right away even though you just ate three hours ago. But, real starvation doesn't work that way. It is estimated that a lean human being can survive up to a month or so without a bite of solid food (provided they have an ample water supply). An obese person can survive *much* longer by burning their fat stores until they are exhausted. But, when the drugs are this powerful (as is the case with the "drugs" in the simple Dorito chip, believe it or not), the brain, completely distracted and motivated only by the effect, wins out over your own better judgment. This is in the very same way the heroin addict loses the battle to the addiction again and again and again... Even though "we don't want to" or "we know better," we regularly rationalize it away as being "just this once" or "only a handful." That's your chemically duped brain talking. You *really do know better*. But you are being controlled. Please never underestimate the power of the foods in control right now. They got ya. No doubt. And right now, they hold all the cards.

But, you are not going to storm their castle all at once, as other paleo plans would have you do. You are far too weak for that at this stage in the grand battle plan. You will be going into "ninja" mode. You are going to infiltrate the castle's defenses very gradually and stealthily. They will never know you're there in the midst of their devious activities. You will take them down one by one by one...

It will probably be sound advice for you to not tell anyone, other than those who can truly sympathize with your efforts, just what it is that you are doing and why. At least not until you start to see some results for yourself. *Paleo*, for as great as the lifestyle is for those who have gotten there, has also received a lot of *bad press* since it came onto the scene. Your very own USDA hates the movement very much, to be sure, as it represents a demonizing of everything that fills their collective wallets. Namely, the giant profits from the agri-businesses of subsidized corn, soy and wheat farming which they ultimately and completely control. Other critics you'll encounter will include those who still cling to the antiquated and debunked low-fat, high-carb sales pitch because anything else just wouldn't be "heart healthy."

Please remember that if you must field a charge against your endeavors such as "everyone in America eats this way; why are you trying to be so different?" rest assured that the claim itself does not represent a strong argument whatsoever against the clear benefits of a paleo eating style. It doesn't even address it. It simply illustrates a sad sheep mentality and a refusal to defy mainstream convention. And, perhaps too great of a love for Hot Pockets. Recall that obesity and diabetes rates are at an all-time high in America, the very worst of all nations with regard to such, and ever-climbing. New research from many fields of science link these rates *directly* to the flawed national diet recommendations over the past 7 decades and to the millions of well-meaning individuals who have blindly followed them ever since. Don't fall for the logic. An opinion held by a majority, no matter how vast that majority may be, is still just an opinion. These opinions of the USDA that became such doctrine but led so many astray were supposedly backed by scientific data. Oops! But, no matter, you are no longer a sheep, you are a ninja.

As far as utilizing the five parts of this section goes, this is where things really need to be taken at your own pace. Habit replacement is difficult as hell and when addictions are connected it becomes that much harder. It's not a race. Nobody is timing you. You can't be in a hurry to break the next addiction on the list. Wait until you are unmistakably clear from the grip of the previous one. At an absolute bare minimum, I would give yourself 21 days before taking on each new addiction in this section. Even a single day less and you're not doing it right. The alarm will go off, your ninja tactics will be exposed, the castle guards will arrest you and the whole campaign will go up in smoke. I am being dramatic but, the truth is, we just don't know how long it will really take to break each of these food addictions. Your body will tell you when it is recovered and ready to move on. But, it surely will not be before 21 days has elapsed. So don't be tempted.

As I already mentioned, but it bears repeating, you're not *trying* to lose weight (even though that will start to become a perceptible byproduct of your efforts the further you get into this program). You are breaking addictions. Back off the scale. In fact, sell the damn scale at your next yard sale.

If you've never read an ingredient label on food you have purchased, it is time you got started. The U.S. government hasn't gotten much right with our food over the years but requiring an ingredient label on everything consumable (that is, *processed* and consumable) has been the very best gift they have brought us thus far, to be certain. Food labels will become your best friend and your guide for where you are headed in the coming parts of this book dealing with addictions. These parts will define for you what it is you are avoiding and all of the clever names it goes by. You'll be surprised at how tactfully our adversaries continually attack us. Eventually, you'll be eating nearly everything fresh. So, labels will lose their importance to us. Single ingredient foods don't need a label.

One last thought, before you get started. Don't forget to use your own best judgment in creating your own personal plan as you progress. I like beets. Beets are super good for you. Well, guess what? It just won't really matter one bit to you just how healthy beets are if *you* can't stand beets. Fortunately, your body will never be starved of nutrients once you have fully adopted a paleo-style plan so *guilting* yourself into eating beets will never become necessary.

PART I: YOUR ADDICTION TO GLUTEN

Are you so done with seeing all of the gluten-free options on your store shelves? If your city is anything like mine, then you have had entire aisles in your mega-super grocery stores taken away and replaced with nothing but gluten-free options. They have some nerve, you've decided.

"What in the hell is gluten anyway?"

"Why did you take away my store aisles and fill them with gluten-free stuff?"

"I don't have celiac disease."

"Isn't that discrimination?"

Gluten is, by definition, a protein composite found in several types of grains. Most notably found in all types of wheat, it is also found in rye and barley.

And guess what? It's bad. It gets its very own chapter all to itself. But, I'll get to why it's bad in a moment.

Made up of two proteins, *gliadin* and *glutenin*, it is the gliadin in gluten which is responsible for the springy, elastic composition of bread and pizza doughs. Without it, your local pizza shop would not be twirling dough over their heads. But it is also this gliadin to which so many react adversely.

Gluten is a sneaky ingredient in so many common processed foods that we don't really want to go there right now except to maybe illustrate one brief example. As I was personally going gluten-free, I was most pissed off in learning that there's quite a lot of wheat in the Twizzlers black licorice that I was oh so very fond of at that particular time in my life.

"Shucks!" I said (that's not what I *really* said). *"It's in everything!"*

And it is. But, relax... You're a ninja. You're not storming the castle. It's all good.

However, none of these musings really matter right now. What matters most is that by that starting with gluten, the very first item to be added on your excluded foods list, you can make a change in the way you eat that will not only be incredibly beneficial in the long-term but will also be only minimally upsetting to your current way of eating. This is primarily due to all of the options to be found on that aisle that you despise so much in your local mega-super grocery store.

But, what is the problem with gluten? There are really two main problems with gluten.

#1 is its toxicity to the human body.

And this means EVERY human body, celiac sufferer or not. Nobody is dealing with gluten very well in spite of what they might tell you. Call it *gluten sensitivity, gluten intolerance* or, the most advanced adverse reaction to gluten, *celiac disease*, it still doesn't matter to me. Look up the numbers. If that many people across the nation can be affected by a food, maybe it's time to stop living on that food. And, believe me, Americans are *living* on gluten. It's everywhere and all are affected by it. You can't tell me otherwise. Even if a person can't be diagnosed with a hint of a single symptom known to derive from gluten consumption, they are still eating a fattening food (the gluten itself isn't necessarily fattening, but it is only ever found in fattening dishes or alcohol). Simple logic says our bodies aren't designed to carry extra weight in the form of perverse amounts of fat cells. Disease always ensues. Therefore, we aren't meant to consume wheat products because they make us fat. If that logic isn't enough for you then I'll just simply ask "do you want to be fat?" I don't. Obesity kills. Diabetes is horrible and a known diet-related problem. Anyone who eats gluten is affected by it in that they are chronically eating a known human toxin whether they "feel" bad or not.

#2 is its prevalence within our food supply.

This is the scary part, my little ninja. But don't be scared.

This is where you'll need to get savvy in reading food labels. Even if your local grocery store doesn't have a gluten-free aisle (or better yet, several aisles), gluten-free products are usually easy to spot. The craze has made food producers so eager to spell out the fact that their brand is gluten-free that you won't have to read the fine print to see if the product fits the bill. It will be clear as day on the front of the package.

On the other hand, there is no requirement for food producers to provide any additional labeling (beyond the standard required label which all processed food products must include) if their product does, in fact, contain gluten. Further, gluten won't typically be listed as such as an ingredient on a food label because it is a *component of its host ingredient*. This would be similar to not listing *protein* in the list of ingredients when chicken is found in a processed food. Sure, it's in there, but it's not listed because it is a *component of the chicken* which is listed. Get it?

Instead, what you are looking for on labels are the crafty disguises that gluten will wear. Look for the following:

Atta (Chapati flour)
Barley (flakes, flour, pearl)
Breading, Bread Stuffing
Brewer's Yeast
Bulgur
Durum (type of wheat)
Einkorn (type of wheat)
Emmer (type of wheat)
Farina
Farro/Faro (also known as Spelt or Dinkel)
Fu (a dried gluten product made from wheat and used in some Asian dishes)
Graham Flour
Hydrolyzed Wheat Protein
Kamut (type of wheat)

Malt, Malt Extract, Malt Syrup, Malt Flavoring
Malt Vinegar
Malted Milk
Matzo, Matzo Meal
Modified Wheat Starch
Oatmeal, Oat Bran, Oat Flour, Whole Oats
Rye
Rye Bread/Flour
Seitan (a meat-like food derived from wheat gluten used in many vegetarian dishes)
Semolina
Spelt (type of wheat also known as Farro, Faro or Dinkel)
Triticale
Wheat
Wheat Bran
Wheat Flour
Wheat Germ
Wheat Starch

Some of the items on this list signal only the *possibility* of gluten being present in the product. However, since you will not have an instrument for either confirming or denying its presence, you will have to avoid all of the list items. You can't take that chance. And, just trust me when I say that, whether it turns out that they contain gluten or not, everything on this list is truly horrible for a human being to consume, and highly addictive. It would be like saying morphine would be great to get hooked on because it isn't heroin.

This list is pretty exhaustive and I trust it. However, when you're at the store, take a moment to plug in the name of the product or the ingredient you are questioning into the internet search on your smart phone this way:

"Is/are _____ gluten-free?"

It works. It is truly an awesome age we are living in.

A good rule of thumb for you to follow during this phase is if it doesn't come from the produce section or the butcher, assume that it contains gluten. Check the label for any of the above list items. And, plug it into an internet search. It's time to get mad and recognize gluten as an enemy inside the castle walls that has had a large hand in the way you have been feeling. It must be eliminated in all its forms. Be relentless in pursuing the bastard.

Make sure you check all processed food items for these ingredients. This includes even those products touted as gluten-free. The standards for labeling foods as gluten-free do not necessarily recognize all of the items on this list of addictive ingredients so don't trust the labels.

I read back what I have written so far and I don't see anywhere where I might have said that this project for personal health that you are taking on was going to be *easy.* It won't be easy. Adapting to the new foods as replacements for your staples will take faithful persistence. I think I only said *you won't go hungry.*

We haven't even looked at what you will be adding in as replacements for these ingredients yet. So don't panic. However, as I get to revealing more of the things that must also be eradicated in this addiction-breaking phase of the program, keep in mind that I am not necessarily replacing them with something that would be considered healthier. In many cases the replacement won't be any more healthy in a broader sense because it will be every bit as fattening as the former product. But it won't contain gluten. You are simply dealing with food addiction #1—*gluten*—at this point. Weight loss won't likely be a side effect you can measure just yet.

Additionally, despite what I said earlier about trusting your body to tell you when an addiction is broken, your transition to gluten-free eating may not be accompanied by feeling better in any way. Mine did. And yours *should.* But don't be discouraged if you don't feel anything until you are a few addictions into this addiction-breaking process. It will happen. Remember how powerful your adversaries are. If you don't feel any change, just be sure to give every addiction at least 21 days and you should be fine to move on.

Assume that all beer contains gluten. It is typically made from barley or wheat, both of which contain gluten. There are gluten-free beer options and they will be labeled accordingly. Hard cider doesn't have gluten and neither does wine. There, you can still drown your sorrows as you lament your food losses. However, alcohol consumption tends to lead to binging and poor judgment. Keep this in mind always. Such an episode for me led to the discovery that Twizzlers black licorice is made from wheat.

"Shucks!"

The discovery was made after I read the empty package on the floor next to my bed the next morning.

If there was anything I could say at this stage in the program that should carry more weight than anything else I could say, it is this. A drug addict, when they are sealed away in a rehab center, can't usually talk a caretaker into getting them a "hit." That would be pretty counter-productive on the part of the rehab center. That's why the patient is sealed away in the first place—to prohibit them access to their fix. An addict must become 100% clean, forever. If not, they never rehabilitated and are still hooked. There really is no such thing as re-rehabilitation. For you, that means that you have to buy into this program wholeheartedly for it to work. I am very sorry but this plan does not allow *cheat* days when it comes to addictive foods. A fully rehabilitated, formerly chronic alcoholic can NEVER say to themselves *"ah, just one rum toddy. It's Christmas!"*

If you slip up and you know you slipped up, be honest with yourself. Start the 21-day clock over again and again until you can make it a permanent change. Don't be discouraged. This is tricky stuff. Dust your ninja outfit off and get back over that wall.

When you reach 21 days it should be a piece of cake to say goodbye to gluten forever.

Put the cake down. I didn't mean that literally.

Before we start looking at suitable replacement products for this first addiction of yours, let's talk about one more thing—dining out. If you frequent fast food establishments and are not accustomed to preparing your own meals, your road to living without gluten will be paved with boulders. This isn't to say you can't travel down this road, it just means the ride is likely to get a bit bumpy.

Because the gluten-free craze has caught on so fiercely in this country, restaurants have almost been forced to create gluten-free menu items at the risk of losing customers. What they haven't been *regulated* to do however is provide you with ingredient labels on their offerings. This leaves determining if you really want to eat it or not completely up to you. You can ask what's in it, but most fast food staff members wouldn't have the faintest idea just what in the hell it is you're talking about when it comes to the list of toxic ingredients listed earlier. So good luck with that. The better option is to become incredibly familiar with every one of the list items for yourself. Figure out the type of processed food products in which each item is most commonly going to be found. You will have to do a little research online and at your local grocery store to do so, but isn't returning you back to optimum health and gaining back your six-pack abs worth it? When you have done so, you can almost eliminate the possibility of gluten contamination by using your deductive reasoning. You have to be on your toes if you really want to eliminate gluten from your diet while dining out. A side of vegetables seems harmless enough but what if that side dish comes with a cream or cheese sauce? Do you know what is used as a thickening agent for sauces of any kind in most restaurants? Wheat flour. Tell your wait staff that you have a severe allergy to gluten and ask for a list of all ingredients from the cook/chef. They should most certainly oblige as nothing inspires restaurant staff more than the word "allergy." If this seems like a pain in the ass to you, the alternative is to not eat out. This is the *very best* option of all.

Once you've truly become gluten free, your favorite restaurants may lose their appeal altogether. Chances are that indulgent dish that you can't wait to devour at your favorite joint is loaded with gluten. And while restaurants have tended to be begrudgingly compliant with the trend by each creating gluten-free menus, most of them haven't put much time or effort into creating one with exciting options on it. Steamed frozen veggies and plain boneless chicken breasts are common fare on these menus. Woo hoo!! No thanks. I can do that at home and it wouldn't cost me $12.95. And, I would use *fresh* vegetables.

Now we can begin to talk about acceptable substitutes for everything that needs to be purged from your pantry during this phase of the plan. Keep in mind that, because gluten has become so vastly spread throughout our food supply, this becomes no small undertaking. *You will feel this* in a very real way and you will need to be prepared for the uncomfortable reality of the changeover. Do it when you're determined to beat the addiction and not just looking to "try it out." Just trying it out would be a bad move. It won't work. I guarantee it. Do it suddenly at a predetermined date and never look back. You should start to feel changes within the first week—some positive and some that might make you feel miserable, but stick with it. The bad gets better. And always remember that 21 days is not the goal for you in eating gluten-free. *Permanent removal of gluten from your life is.* 21 days is just the marker we use for the green light for tackling the next addiction on the list.

Never forget that the enemy of this phase will do its very best to make you feel like your body "needs" gluten once you rid yourself of it. It's a lie. Don't fall for it. You have to will yourself with the "want-to" to survive each of these phases.

Remember what I said about the gliadin in gluten which gives pizza crust its desirable spongy consistency? Well, sadly, gluten-free food science hasn't duplicated this consistency in any of its pizza flours as of this writing. I also will not lie to you and say that a peanut butter and jelly sandwich on gluten-free bread rivals the same sandwich made with Wonder bread. It doesn't. And gluten-free pasta sure isn't like Grandma's.

But you won't go hungry.

That is my promise.

So where are you most likely to find gluten? Anywhere you'd find wheat. Obvious gluten hangouts are bread, buns, rolls, cakes, pies, pizza, pasta and pretzels. But, as I stated earlier, wheat shows up in so many things that aren't so obvious. Thickened sauces and candy were the two that opened my eyes the widest and made me realize that I can never assume the best in my processed food choices. On this plan, your food choices have to be scrutinized diligently by someone who is educated on where to find gluten and determined to avoid it in any of its many forms at all costs. That someone has to be you. You can't trust anyone, including your own government, to do it properly for you.

Your grocery store may have the gluten-free aisle or aisles I talked about earlier and it may not. But, it is likely that the same choices are also found next to the foods they are a gluten-free option for. For example, there are probably gluten-free pasta noodles mixed right in with regular toxic noodles on the normal pasta aisle of your local store. My suggestion, since this is such a new frontier for you, is to get familiar with the layout of your favorite store and if they don't have enough gluten-free choices to satisfy you in this early phase of your return to health, then find a new store to shop at that does. If you are in an incredibly rural and remote area, Amazon.com will ship all of the gluten-free staples you can imagine right to your front door. We can't let a perceived unavailability of gluten-free choices be an excuse for not taking this very first step in the rehabilitation process.

Don't forget to examine the ingredient list of anything processed for the toxic ingredients listed earlier. *Even if the packaging says gluten-free!*

OK, so here we go. Again, you will not be replacing unhealthy foods with healthier options in this phase. On the contrary, most of these aren't any more nutritive than the foods you're eliminating. Neither are they "diet" foods. They are simply not as toxic as gluten and, more importantly, these replacements are not known to be nearly as addictive.

Below is a list of flours commonly used in the processing of gluten-free products. As long as you see any of these as main ingredients rather than the bad guys listed earlier, you are good to go with them during this first addiction breaking phase. Hopefully, the lack of taste and consistency in these replacements will eventually inspire you to give up all of these types of foods altogether rather than long to return to the ones that used to taste good to you.

Amaranth Flour
Arrowroot Flour
Banana Flour
Brown Rice Flour
Buckwheat Flour
Chia Flour
Chickpea (Garbanzo) Flour
Coconut Flour
Corn Flour
Corn Meal
Hemp Flour
Lupin Flour
Maize Flour
Millet Flour
Potato Flour
Potato Starch Flour
Quinoa Flour
Sorghum Flour
Soya Flour
Tapioca Flour
Teff Flour
White Rice Flour

Also, be on the lookout for gluten-free pasta alternatives made from legumes such as black beans and kidney beans. These are one-ingredient foods which are far superior nutritionally to pastas made from gluten-free alternative flours. And as far as taste and texture go, these were my personal favorites during the time I spent in this phase of the eating plan.

If you are a baker, you stand a better chance of *creating* gluten-free items that will satisfy you over finding them on your store shelves. Being a baker you will also quickly notice the inferiority of non-wheat flour as a baking ingredient. Ah well, it's for the greater good of your overall health.

Now is the time to start your list of excluded foods. Create a document which will list all of the foods being eliminated during this phase. It can be as simple as writing down the word "gluten." For a one-word entry like this to work though, you must know, without question, what foods this pertains to. And that is *all of them*, every single last one. A better strategy is to write down broader terms on your list, such as bread, buns, flour tortillas, licorice, etc.

Stick with the program no matter what once you start this first phase. Again, this isn't just taking a break from gluten, you are ridding yourself of it forever, so be ready mentally for the psychological assault that will follow. Because this is an addiction to a substance your body and mind have tricked you into repeatedly providing for them, the process of suddenly depriving yourself of it can't be taken lightly. The two most effectively employed tactics your body will use against you to get more gluten are light-headedness and the sensation of extreme hunger pangs. There are more you might experience but these two are gripping. No lie. But, with effort, you will become released from the hook of gluten and these will disappear. At least until the next addiction breaking campaign is undertaken. You will have to outlast these withdrawal symptoms to win this phase. If you stumble, go back to day one as I stressed before and give it a more focused attempt.

You can always take a break before starting the next addiction phase. Take the time to rest up and mentally prepare yourself for the next round now that you know more of what to expect. Just don't celebrate breaking your addiction to gluten with a jelly donut.

PART II: YOUR ADDICTION TO SUGAR

Congratulations!

If you have made it this far then you have lasted at least 21 days through the first addiction breaking cycle in this program without having a bite of gluten-containing food. You should feel a sense of accomplishment knowing that you have beaten the withdrawal symptoms that go along with gluten addiction. That feat is not an easy one. And it should fire you up for this next phase because you are going to need all of the extra strength that you can muster right now to be completely honest.

I know it wasn't comfortable and I know substitutes for wheat-based products suck. However, I am guessing that you feel a little "cleaner" inside and that you may have experienced some positive body changes to go along with all of the ones that may have made you feel quite uncomfortable. It is my hope, this early into the process of cleaning up the food addictions that have a hold over you, that already you can start to see how powerful the wrong types of food for the human body can truly be. This revelation should be enough to inspire you to never feel inclined to ingest anything containing gluten ever again.

Now onto a much more difficult stage in food addiction reversal—the elimination of sugar. Sugar, in all of its many sneaky variations, can be assumed to be included as an ingredient in just about any food product manufactured worldwide. Gluten may be prominent in our processed food supply, but *sugar is everywhere*. It is absolutely inescapable unless a conscious campaign is waged to become educated on how to avoid it. This is what you'll be doing in this next battle in the war on food addiction.

"Do I really have to give up sugar?"

Only if you want to live a healthful and energized life. You really won't miss it once you get there, I absolutely promise this to you.

So why is sugar so bad? Do I really need to spell this out? You have been conditioned on the evils of sugar since your mother first told you it is bad for your teeth. And the mouth is just the gatekeeper for the rest of the body. She was right. Sugar not only viciously attacks that first area of the body as it passes through but it does egregious harm everywhere else it goes. Let's take a look at some of the reasons that sugar is so toxic to the human body.

1.) There is absolutely no nutritive value to be derived from most types of sugar. Zero. It is not needed in any form by the body and can actually be produced inside the body instead (in the form of glucose) from other food sources and burned as fuel, if prompted to do so. This is not an obvious *detriment* of sugar consumption. However, as I will expand on a little further in a moment, for any sugars that do happen to have some nutritive value, their nutrients will not be in enough abundance to justify the bodily harm they will also cause.
2.) Most added sugar in processed foods is predominately fructose. Fructose is metabolized in the liver and much of it is stored in the body as fat in the case of excess, which isn't difficult to achieve considering the extreme amounts of fructose that are present in processed foods.
3.) Body regulation of the hormone insulin, which controls the processing of glucose in the bloodstream, is hampered by excess sugar consumption. Repeated patterns of excess sugar consumption cause the cells to become less and less affected by insulin production. This is a condition known as insulin resistance and is a leading indicator of future problems such as metabolic syndrome, cardiovascular disease and type II diabetes.
4.) Studies have shown that persons who consume large daily amounts of sugar are at a much higher risk for most types of cancer than those who do not. I will interject my own opinion here based on what I consider common sense. If you were to do a little research on cancer—how it appears, how it lives, how it thrives—you will find that it feeds on sugar, exclusively. In fact, this relationship with sugar is so necessary for the survival of cancer cells that, as soon as the supply of sugar to these cells ceases, they die. Says a lot, doesn't it? This fact is mostly hidden from the public for whatever reason. I have my theories as to why but that would be for another day. Need a cure for cancer? Quit eating sugar. There you go. It's been there all along and yet no

one shouts it from the rooftops because it wasn't discovered in a lab and, therefore, would not be in the running for Nobel Prize consideration. It just wouldn't be considered the *miracle cure* that everyone seems to be searching for. Please understand that I am not saying that all forms of cancer are suddenly able to be cured by stopping sugar ingestion. I have no research of my own to back this up. Once formed, cancer cells don't follow predictable life stages. However, I am convinced that, in a cancer-free body, most cancers are *preventable* by keeping added sugar to very reasonable levels. Again, this is just my opinion based on simple reasoning through the typical behavior and life cycle of cancer cells. I am not a doctor. I am not trying to cure cancer.

5.) Just like addictive drugs, sugar stimulates dopamine release in the reward center of the brain. This is the physiological effect of sugar consumption to which people become addicted and which makes ceasing consumption of it so hard to accomplish.

Sugar comes in many forms and is disguised by many names. Food labels are required to list the amount of *sugars* (in grams) that a food product contains per serving. This reading can come from any of a number of sources of added sugar. None of them are any good whatsoever. There is no acceptable quantity (in grams) of sugar that could be listed on a label. If there is any amount other than 0g shown next to *sugars* on a label, you can count on the fact that your body will expend an unreasonable amount of resources to process that substance through your body. The side effects of which will be enormous but quite possibly undetected by you because you have become so accustomed to them. Let's look at some sources of sugars on a food label.

Agave Syrup
Brown Sugar
Cane Sugar
Corn Sweetener
Corn Syrup
Corn Syrup Solids
Dextrose
Evaporated Cane Juice
Fructose

Fruit Juice Concentrate
Galactose
High Fructose Corn Syrup
Honey (yes, honey)
Sucrose
Lactose
Malt Syrup
Maltose
Maple Syrup
Molasses
Raw Sugar
Turbinado Sugar
Table Sugar
White Sugar

Again, these are but *some* of the more common ways in which sugar could be listed on a food label. There are really close to 100 or more ways it actually could also be spelled out. But, you're not going to exhaust yourself searching for it in an ingredient list. Instead, you should only concern yourself with the gram content of *sugars* from the Nutrition Facts section of the labels you inspect. If it is greater than 0g, it's not an approved food choice for this phase of ridding yourself of your addiction to sugar.

Nutrition Facts

Serving Size (83g)
Servings Per Container

Amount Per Serving

Calories 280   Calories from Fat 180

	% Daily Value*
Total Fat 21g	**32%**
Saturated Fat 13g	**65%**
Trans Fat 0g	
Cholesterol 0mg	**0%**
Sodium 115mg	**5%**
Total Carbohydrate 25g	**8%**
Dietary Fiber 4g	**16%**
Sugars 19g	
Protein 2g	

This phase of this program almost precludes dining out whatsoever. Think about how much effort and care you put into your food choices during the previous phase of going gluten-free. Unfortunately, there is no real way to truly know what is being put into your food out of your sight. Gluten was relatively easy to ask about at a restaurant, sugar is not. And because sugar is even more powerful and destructive than gluten, you can't risk contaminating your efforts with sugar you didn't know was added to your food. Please heed my advice and make dining out *completely prohibited* during this phase. Conditioning yourself to avoid dining out right now will also make the act of dining out itself much less appealing as you learn how to eat only from your approved list down the road. And that's a good thing. Dining out is social and I get its appeal but it's no way to regularly abide by this new way of eating/living that you have agreed to take on.

I should be very clear about something before we continue. I don't eat the things that I could be recommending that you use as replacements for sugar during this phase of cleansing. They are not good for you. But neither is sugar. Some say they could be worse for you than sugar. Some say otherwise. But these have all been long eliminated from my diet and added to my excluded list. And they will eventually wind up on your excluded list as well. I am talking about artificial sweeteners.

How could I possibly recommend aspartame over natural raw sugar?

"The nerve!" you say.

That is certainly not what I am saying at all. Please hear me when I say that I don't recommend aspartame to anyone for any reason whatsoever. If you absolutely cannot be without something sweet at a given moment, the only two choices for sugar substitutes I would ever refer you to are coconut sugar (or coconut nectar—a liquid form of it) and stevia. These are not really *artificial* sweeteners at all but are rather completely natural alternatives to table sugar. At the time of this writing, no studies exist revealing any dangers in human consumption of these two sweeteners. The same cannot be said about any of the other alternative artificial sweeteners on the market such as aspartame, sucralose and saccharin. Does this make coconut sugar and stevia safe because there are no negative reports out about them yet? Not hardly.

Know that I am only recommending these two sweeteners in the case of emergency, when it might be the only way to keep you from a Ding-Dong. For the heavy sugar-laden soda drinker, the only alternative which will register 0g under *sugars* in the Nutrition Facts section of the soda label will most likely be a diet soda drink that contains aspartame. If this is your only means of steering clear of sugar, *drink at your own peril* but get off soda of all kinds as quickly as you possibly can. Aspartame is proven to be deadly and debilitating. The exact same can be said of sugar. Sodas are typically sweetened with one or the other so there aren't really any *good* sodas. But, there are better sodas that are now being sweetened with stevia that are fairly new on the market. So, make these your first choice if you are able to. And then be done with soda altogether.

And let's be clear, fruit juice is a horrible replacement for soda. It's no better at all in spite of its "healthy" reputation.

Wait a minute, so why shouldn't you use honey or raw sugar or 100% fruit juice as a replacement for table sugar? They are all natural, right? This is *somewhat* true, based on how truthfully the processing of each type of "natural" sugar may be reported to us. But, this logic also assumes some form of nutritive value being assigned to these "healthy" substitutes in order to make them a better choice. The truth is, there is *some* nutritive value to be found in each one, but it isn't enough to invalidate the harm that they, just like table sugar, also cause. Additionally, fruit juice, which logically seems like the best substitute, contains sugar which is so ridiculously concentrated that even a relatively small serving of it presents massive quantities of sugar which would never be encountered naturally from just eating fruit.

So can you not eat fruit during this phase either?

Actually, no. But, before you accuse this program of being the worst eating plan since the Atkin's New Diet Revolution, let's talk about the glycemic index and how different sugar-filled foods can create a type of recurring pendulum effect in our bodies and why this reaction to sugar can be so dangerous for us.

The glycemic index of foods is basically a measurement of the capacity of a carbohydrate to influence blood sugar levels. There is a lot of broad science behind these measurements and the exact precision of the calculations involved is debatable, but overall, the metric can be used somewhat reliably to decide which foods to eat. It's pretty easy. Low-glycemic foods, such as vegetables, fruit and meat (with a glycemic index ranking of 55 or less) are preferable to high-glycemic foods like pasta, bread and candy (with a glycemic index ranking of 70 or more). Without delving into a lot of hard science, the process essentially occurs this way. High-glycemic foods are almost instantly transformed into glucose and assimilated into the bloodstream, spiking the levels of glucose present in the blood at that time. This is also associated with and felt as a rise in body energy levels. When blood sugar content resumes a more normal reading, energy levels slow in the other direction resulting in a crash of energy levels. Low-glycemic foods, on the other hand, are processed more slowly without an immediate transference into glucose. With this slower release into the bloodstream, the body stays in a steady state of performance without experiencing extreme highs and lows in energy levels.

Insulin, the glucose-regulating hormone the body uses to process the foods it is fed, is secreted by the pancreas and maintained in a healthy body within a very narrow range of fluctuations in production levels. This insulin is the mechanism by which glucose enters the blood. Low-glycemic foods do not usually trigger insulin secretion. High-glycemic foods, on the other hand, are the ones that drive insulin production in the body. However, constant cycles of insulin secretion and cessation of secretion that are *directly relative to food choices* are not desirable for a normal human being. This represents an excessive load on the regulating organs of the liver, pancreas and kidneys and can lead to a host of negative metabolic conditions. This affects just about everybody eating a mainly processed food diet at every meal. Not to mention the fact that these cycles, driven by high-glycemic foods, lead to excess fat storage.

Now back to fruit. Since this phase is a cleanse from sugar and a recovery from the effects that sugar has had on your body for as long as it has been allowed to be a major component of the foods you eat, fruit must also be considered sugar for now. The sugar in fruit is not recognized any differently by your body than the sugar in a Snickers bar. The difference between them lies in the way that your body *processes the sugar* in fruit. This has to do mainly with fruit's fiber content. Studies have shown that the fiber in fruit slows digestion and can prevent the spike in blood sugar levels that would occur from the introduction of the same amount of sugar from a substance, such as a candy bar, without the naturally occurring fiber. This phenomenon is what causes fruit to be ranked low on the glycemic index. Fruit also has great stores of vitamins and nutrient content that a Snickers bar could only dream of. However, it is very possible during this sugar detox phase, that the sugar in fruit could very easily cause cravings for more sugar that will make this phase that much more difficult for you. You can have fruit back soon. Hang in there.

So we have talked a bit about some of what is eliminated from our plate in this phase of addiction eradication. What is left? Not much it would seem. But, press on. You don't even know how good this will be for your overall health. It will be worth some discomfort to get there.

Because, it is the spike and the consequent crash of blood sugar levels that we are trying to limit for ourselves during this and future phases, the absence of irregular body energy levels will be the indicator for us that we are doing things right. If your body energy levels don't even out and you still find yourself experiencing radical highs and lows once you've begun this phase, chances are that you are encountering hidden sugar from a source you will need to discover for yourself and eliminate. If this is the case, start the 21-day clock over at the point this discovery is made and corrected. Although, be aware that it is very possible that heavy starch consumption could also be the culprit in these blood glucose fluctuations. Since starch isn't condemned at this point in the program, carry on if you find that it (rather than sugar) is responsible for the peaks and valleys. But, make an effort now to eat starch more sparingly than you have previously.

You will be very discouraged by the labels you will be reading during this phase. When I said earlier that everything has sugar in it, that is a literal fact when it comes to processed food. If processed foods comprise most, if not all, of your daily menu, then you will really need to abandon the microwave and turn to the stove in order to be successful in eliminating sugar from your diet. Get out (and dust off) the cook books and start preparing your own meals. Small meals with few ingredients are best to start with if you are not accustomed to cooking for yourself. Anywhere a recipe calls for sugar you will use stevia or coconut sugar. Make sure you don't forget that you're also done with gluten permanently so substitute any (wheat) flour a recipe calls for with one of the approved substitutes from the last chapter. Meal preparation is not that difficult. It is just a habit that needs to be developed. You will get better at it with each meal you prepare and you will also find that a prepared meal with fresh ingredients tastes so much better than a processed one. If you are encouraged by your progress through this program so far, use that as motivation to begin cooking for yourself. As I said before, succeeding through the rest of this program depends on it.

This particular phase of the program is by far the toughest to get through because you aren't just eliminating *added* sugar, you are eliminating all sugar for 21 days in order to fully detoxify yourself from sugar's ill effects. Some things (besides fruit) that have naturally occurring sugar that will be sorely missed during these 21 days are milk, most milk products (excluding fermented products such as most cheeses and heavy whipping cream; check the Nutrition Facts section of the label for these to make sure they're at 0g for sugars), tomatoes (also a fruit) and tomato based sauces. Although this phase seems extremely limiting, there will be plenty to eat. If processed and fast food are common meals for you, this phase can feel almost unbearable at times. But it's only 21 days and then many things get returned to your pantry.

Now is the time to get creative with your eating habits. Nothing other than conditioning through tradition says human beings need to eat three meals a day. Or, every 2-3 hours as is the habit of many due to "expert" reports suggesting such. Meals don't need to have an entree, two sides and a dessert. Our conditioning says that sautéed broccoli by itself isn't a meal. The truth is, when you make it through these first two addiction breaking phases, you have eliminated the two most craving-inducing food substances known to man—grain products and sugar. Your conditioning will become less meaningful to you because your hunger should start to diminish. This is because your cravings will start to diminish. You may not notice it right away but you won't be hungry nearly as often as you were prior to committing to this program. And it just may be that sautéed broccoli all by itself becomes one of your favorite meals. It is one of mine, to be sure. And, by the way, once you really get going with this second phase, *if you're not hungry, don't eat*. These are new words for you to live by every single day. Don't prepare something to eat just because it's "lunch time." Get rid of your destructive habits of conditioning.

It truly is a fantastic feeling to have sustained energy throughout each day with hunger for the next meal that occurs only mildly (without the searing hunger pangs you were previously accustomed to). If you follow my instructions closely, you will feel both effects by the time the 21 days are up for this phase. But, one of the most encouraging results of this new eating program of yours is that you will be *eating less*. Grain and sugar cravings incite us to eat much larger portions of foods at each sitting than we would normally eat. You will become satisfied with much less food once you are through each of these first two phases. This is exactly why weight loss will be an inevitable byproduct of this program. You will start see a difference in your body composition before these 21 days are elapsed. I guarantee it. But I still don't want you to step on the scale. Weight loss is not what we're striving for yet.

Some of the things that will become your go-to foods (in order to make it through this phase) are meats, eggs, cheeses (with 0g sugars only), seafood, vegetables, nuts, legumes, alternative flours and fermented foods (such as pickles and sauerkraut). Eat these in any quantities you'd like during these 21 days.

Anything labeled "sugar-free" at the grocery store is not recommended whatsoever to help you endure this phase. I am trying to get you accustomed to real food; fresh food that is prepared by you. I can't stop you from them but let me just warn you that anything labeled "sugar-free" will be filled with all of those horrible chemicals designed to replicate the sweetness of sugar. They also produce cravings and will make staying away from sugar next to impossible. Additionally, many of the artificial sweeteners used most commonly in our food supply will mess with insulin production and create spikes in blood glucose leading to energy peaks and dips and a whole host of other problems. This is in spite of the 0g reading under sugars on the Nutrition Facts section of their labels. Do yourself a favor and skip the sugar-free ice cream. Go to bed already.

If you have to have *something* sweet, seek out (or make) something sweetened with stevia or coconut sugar before turning to anything else sweetened with aspartame, sucralose, or saccharin. And make sure whatever it is reads 0g under sugars in the Nutrition Facts. Coconut sugar does not read 0g under sugars, by the way. But, we're giving it a pass because it ranks very low on the glycemic index. And because it isn't a deadly chemical.

I used sugar-free gum sweetened with xylitol (a sugar alcohol which I will talk about in a later chapter) from my local health food market quite effectively to beat my cravings for sugar during this phase. Sometimes it isn't food your body is craving. It is more sugar. This gum trick works wonders to give it what it thinks it wants.

For those sugary cereal junkies who are not liking this program at all right now, I am sorry. Fry up some bacon and eggs and add some stevia to your morning coffee (heavy whipping cream also has 0g of sugars) and you'll be good to go. Or chew some gum sweetened with xylitol.

Start skipping meals during this phase. Train your body to go longer between feedings. You will not die. Drink water when you're hungry—it has a hunger-calming effect. Distract yourself with something active. Watching TV is not active and is an awful activity to occupy yourself with when you're hungry. Television commercials pitching processed foods will wreak havoc on your will to press on through the discomfort of this phase. Limit or eliminate the activity of TV watching altogether if at all possible.

I am not saying don't eat when you're hungry. I am saying try very hard to make certain it's really a *need for food* that your body is sending you signals for and not just a craving for something it is still hooked on before you oblige the urge.

Best of luck in completing this phase of the program. It will all be downhill for you as you continue past these 21 days. Your body will be cleaned up of the two worst health-sabotaging culprits in our food supply and you will be feeling great and completely undeterred from your goal of a truly 100% paleo-inspired lifestyle.

At this point, you can either add the one-word entry of *sugar* to your excluded list or take the time to write out everything that used to tempt you that you've now discovered has sugar in it. But remember that your exclusions from this chapter also include all of the artificial sweeteners we discussed as well. This only leaves stevia and coconut sugar (or coconut nectar) in the case of emergency.

In the next chapter we will still be adding to your excluded list but you will have cleared the two highest hurdles to success in this program. The new exclusions will be easy for you.

PART III: YOUR ADDICTION TO STARCHES

You did it! You are really home free at this point. The really grueling part of regaining your health and returning to an optimal body weight is done. This is the point where all of your ninja efforts have nearly served their purpose. You now have a stronghold inside the castle. You can take off your ninja suit and enjoy the fruits (literally) of your labor. Remember, all changes are permanent. Gluten and added sugar are off the table forever. You are adopting a new way of eating altogether. Monitor your excluded list closely and keep it memorized at all times.

Let's talk about *reality* for a moment. Am I to expect that you will never eat gluten or sugar ever again for as long as you live? I hope for your sake that I *can* expect as much. They're nasty and deadly. But that hope may not be realistic. Here's the truth of the matter. Let's say you "accidentally" ate a jelly donut after you have completed these first two parts of the program.

"What do I do?" you ask.

Well you won't die.

And you won't have to go back and start the addiction breaking processes over again because you're not addicted...,

Yet.

You will feel the effects of this slip-up. You will get a "sugar rush" and you will crash. You could get a rash, feel congested, get stomach cramps or just find yourself feeling generally crappy with any of a number of other symptoms related to your accidental overdose of gluten and sugar. You see, once you have rehabilitated completely from gluten and sugar, side effects of them will become way more evident to you than when you were hooked. Your former tolerance of their effects is now gone. My bet is you won't like the consequences of going back to gluten or sugar whatsoever and you will say *"no more jelly donuts for me."*

On the other hand, this is a slippery slope you have found yourself on. Because gluten and sugar are so powerful, it is also very possible that you find yourself screaming down the slope like a bowling ball fired out of a cannon with no hope of stopping until you smash into jagged pieces at the bottom of the ravine.

Just from one jelly donut.

Now, *this* is a different situation. For this kind of psychological collapse, unfortunately, you must go back to the beginning of this book and start all over. Sorry.

I say this is a psychological collapse because it truly is. You have hands to grab food with in order to stuff it into your pie-hole but you can't do it without your brain giving your hands clearance to do so. There just has to be some self-restraint that kicks in when you occasionally screw up your eating habits in order to keep from undoing all the good you've done for yourself. Resist the power of addictive foods to lure you back. This is on you. You need to keep yourself from becoming prone to slipping right back into an addicted state. Some personality types are very prone to addictions, both food addictions and otherwise. They become especially vulnerable to their former addictions when faced with feelings of depression or hopelessness. This is a known fact. Knowledge is power. Use this knowledge proactively (if you feel you might have this type of personality) to your advantage. Looking at the bright side of things, powering through the urge to revert back to your old habits could just take you to a place where you aren't depressed any longer. Especially if that depression was in part due to low self-esteem brought on by discontentment with your own body image or lingering health concerns that just might be corrected by sticking with this lifestyle change.

But the very best strategy of all to avoid these food fiends and the terrible consequence of having to read this book again is to never give them an open door back into your digestive system in the first place.

Don't get me wrong, this is a good read. No doubt about it. But if you ever have to go back and read it again, it means your fix has hooked you again. Damn it, Jim!

Now, we need to talk about *starches*. Starch is a common ingredient in lots of foods from corn to bananas (starch level depends on ripeness) to potatoes. It is also the main component of those alternative flours you have been baking with.

"So you're telling me I'm addicted to bananas?!"

Well, that's not exactly what I'm saying at this point. It's a *maybe*.

Proof of the body's tendency to become addicted to and feel effects from foods other than grain flours and sugar is not really documented anywhere. But, let's go back to the glycemic index for a moment and discuss starches. Most all of them rank above the high marker of 70 on the index. This means they absolutely will fuel a surge in insulin production with all of the resulting side effects.

This is bad.

My justification for believing that there is a potential for addiction to starches of any kind is really a leap of faith based on common sense. Since I can't steer you to any studies on the matter, I will steer you to potato chips.

As I was developing this program, I was eating lots of potato chips made with avocado oil. They had only three ingredients in them—potatoes, avocado oil and salt. Relatively healthy, right? That's what I thought too. Take a look at the ingredient list for regular old potato chips—Lay's or Ruffles, doesn't matter. It's very long and you've barely ever heard of any of the ingredients other than potatoes. Just what are you eating when you eat potato chips, anyway? Scary. This is why potato chips made with just a single healthy oil and salt seemed like such a breakthrough for me at the time. Problem was I was eating them a lot. And I mean *a lot*. Half a bag was my dinner some nights. While I have no scientific evidence to support it, I think I was *addicted to potato chips made with avocado oil*. But, in my estimation, it was really just the starch in the potatoes that was causing the overeating. This is the component in the chips that would have caused the blood sugar spikes and the cravings for more for me.

I believe that foods other than gluten and sugar that raise insulin levels and spike blood glucose *also create cravings and are addictive*. I just don't feel like they are as powerful as gluten and sugar. Sort of like the relationship of marijuana to heroin. They're both addictive but one is usually used in a very recreational manner without really creating a *hooked* effect while the other will take over your mind, consume your soul and control you completely.

One thing is for certain, starches which do raise insulin levels and spike blood glucose will make you fat.

That one isn't my opinion.

In this chapter we are going to look at all of the starches that should be considered for elimination from our diet to permanently take up residence on our excluded list. But, before we start eliminating yet again, how about a bit of good news? It's time we added back in naturally occurring sugars. You can now have your dairy, tomatoes and all your other fruits back. Yahoo!! Please remember to eat these types of foods in much less quantity and frequency than other foods that are not excluded. The sugar in them, naturally occurring or not, can still cause cravings so be careful. We don't want to blow up the whole campaign over an apple. And they can be fattening. So, if weight loss is your goal with this program, go easy on these. Also, please be sure to reintroduce them one at a time to see if they still agree with you. Yes, that is right, they may not be tolerated well by you at all even though you may have previously eaten them like crazy. I talk more about how to conduct this process in the coming paragraphs.

A quick word about dairy products. In the next chapter, we will talk about foods which are *allergenic* (non-fermented dairy is definitely one of them), that is they tend to cause any number of allergic reactions in a much larger cross-section of the population than foods which are considered non-allergenic. But, for now all I would like to say about dairy is to please stay away from low fat and reduced fat dairy products. They are no good. When fat is removed, sugar is added. Keep the fat. Ditch the sugar. Trust me. We will get to the reasoning behind this in later chapters. And obviously, if you're allergic to dairy, for God's sake don't let my giving full fat dairy a green light in this section cause you to start eating dairy products. As you well know, they are toxic for you. I can't change that.

There are a lot of recent studies on certain types of starches that can be categorized as *resistant starches*. These are considered healthier starches which are said to affect blood glucose differently than slowly digested or rapidly digested starches. However, these studies are mostly recent and ultimately incomplete in terms of precisely how this categorization is important to your health and your weight. If you'd like to investigate the subject, do an internet search for "resistant starches" and get ready to swim through the many contradictory reports relating to it. In a nutshell, resistant starches pass through our small intestines untouched, without being digested at all. Yet, in the absence of hard data, I am going to limit our discussion about them. I am not steering you away from resistant starches necessarily. There are great health benefits reported in many studies regarding them. I am saying check things out for yourself.

The basic reality about starches is that, when eaten in abundance, they have the potential to spike blood glucose. This is likely to cause cravings. Cravings will promote weight gain. Lastly, you will be prone to bloating and flatulence from eating too much starch. Let's clear the air here (pun intended), these are all wonderful reasons to limit starches.

Once you have completely rid yourself of gluten and added sugar, food types that remain (including all starches) are best tested through self-experimentation to see if they should be allowed to continue as part of your diet. This is where we are headed here (and in coming chapters) and this is also where your excluded and approved lists will start to deviate a little bit from the lists of everyone else who has gone through this program. This self-testing can produce lists that vary greatly from person to person.

When testing starchy foods, drop certain ones from your regular diet for several weeks and then reintroduce them and see how you feel. Also, see if eating them either slows weight loss or promotes weight gain.

You really do need to cleanse yourself thoroughly from foods you will be testing out going forward. Your body can build up tolerance to certain types of foods, even those you are allergic to. You may not even notice that a food is not tolerated well until you remove it from your diet for a while. Let's set a minimum of 14 days as the standard cleanse duration for foods we test from here on out. This is a complete removal from the diet of the food type in question with the sole intention of reintroduction for the sake of study two weeks later. Don't be confused, this is not the same activity as breaking an addiction.

As you conduct these experiments on yourself, there are certain signs of trouble you should watch for as foods are reintroduced. Some of these are upset stomach (nausea and/or vomiting), cramping, diarrhea and headaches. You could find yourself with simply a vague, unexplained feeling of discontent. You could also see external physical signs such as rashes and skin blotches. But these are not nearly all of the manifestations in which a poor food choice for your body could show up. You know how you felt before you ate it. How do you feel now? The *same* or *better* are the only two gate permits that should allow it back onto your approved list.

Let me also forewarn you that anything consumed can affect you adversely *without* warning signs that you can see or feel necessarily. Your body is very good at taking in all the poisons you might feed it and getting right to work on counteracting the assault all while trying very hard not to alert you to the issue. It seems like it just doesn't want to make a scene about anything until it just can't keep it from you any longer. And then it might be too late for you to do anything about the problem. Often there really are signs but they are missed because they aren't glaringly obvious. Don't eat test foods and wait to feel bad. Instead, eat them and *pay very close attention* for several hours up to several days afterward.

I am really hoping that your daily food intake now consists of markedly smaller portions with much fewer incidence of processed food intake than it did prior to your taking on the task of breaking your gluten addiction. You should also be feeling some overall weight loss by now, be hungry less frequently and you should definitely be working toward preparing all of your own meals. If you have made it this far and all of the above are not the case, then I am sad to report that something has gone horribly awry. You're not doing things right at all with regard to the plan I have laid out so far. If you have really removed gluten and added sugar properly from your diet the result is a grocery store without many processed products available for your consumption. There may very well be no processed food options available at all. That is a good thing rather than the end of the world. Please try to start looking at it that way. You're just that much closer to reaching the goal of this program.

This is a good time to restate that goal. We are working toward eating an exclusively *paleo-inspired diet which does not really encourage processed foods in any form whatsoever for any reason.* Ugh! I know. You're not quite there yet. But don't panic. It's achievable. It does help to talk through it now and again and you have to admit that you're much further along than you were prior to kicking your gluten and sugar habits. As I said before, the hard part is over.

I am going to now assume that weight loss is a primary goal for your reading this book. Such an assumption makes your relationship with starches less friendly than the relationship between starches and a fit triathlete. If you're a fit triathlete and you have no trouble eating starches, skip the rest of this chapter.

The following is a list of starches which tend to rank high on the glycemic index and should be avoided or severely limited (*avoided* is better). And, unfortunately it is also time to get rid of all the alternative flours that were acceptable during your previous phases of addiction breaking. They aren't acceptable anymore. You'll never lose the extra weight you'd like to lose if they are a regular part of your diet.

Bananas (starchy when not fully ripe and loaded with sugar—you definitely won't lose weight with these)

Corn and Corn Products (including hominy)
Legumes (all of them from green peas to peanuts to navy beans; if you're not sure if it's a legume, look it up)
Plantains
Popcorn
Potatoes (red, white, Russet, etc.)
Pumpkin
Rice and Rice Products
Root Vegetables (excluding low-starch varieties like carrots and turnips)
Squash (acorn, butternut, etc.)
Sweet Potatoes (all varieties)

It is common in paleo writings to see regular potatoes condemned while sweet potatoes get promoted as perfectly acceptable. I don't get it. They are so similar in compositional makeup that either they should both be demonized or both be allowed. Don't buy the sweet potato hype. And don't eat either of these until you have reached your target weight. And then eat them only if they agree with you and if you can't help yourself.

This is where I might start to take some heat. Those are healthy things on that list above (for the most part). So, why would I condemn good things to eat?

True, the list is comprised of items that are generally regarded as healthy but my argument is that they are not as *nutrient dense* as a lot of the other food items that remain on your approved list at this point. Oh yeah, and they're also fattening. But, my point is, you will not be losing out on precious vitamins and minerals by deleting some or all of these list items as the nutrients in them will be found in better abundance from other approved food sources.

Broccoli is high in vitamin C and potassium, for example. Let me use that fact to illustrate a point for my critics. It may be argued that by favoring certain foods over others one may become deficient in certain micronutrients their body is in need of. But this is part of the conditioning our government and vitamin manufacturers have subjected us to for decades with their scientifically derived recommended nutrient values. Rather than spark a ton of debate about the subject, my only question is *will this new way of eating be better than your old way?* Don't approach eating scientifically anymore. Ask yourself if too much kale and not enough carrots is better than too many Cheetos and not enough pancakes with sugary syrup? If I eat too much broccoli and not much of anything else will I die from vitamin C and potassium overdose or quite possibly, malnutrition from the lack of other valid nutrients? Come on now. Stop already. Your conditioning needs to go.

When a person is eating the right types of food for their body and they are also freed of all of their food addictions (this is critical), they subconsciously tend to choose foods which have the nutrient makeup their body needs. This nudging by your body will never be as powerful as a craving for an addictive substance; it is subtler than that. It represents a body functioning as nature intended. When you finally feel this happen to you, listen to the urging. Your body is way more reliable in telling you what it needs than your government is. It isn't always so that what your body is suggesting at any particular moment will even be available to you, but it's nice to know that you have a new authority on the subject to listen to. On the other hand, if your body is hankering for Hot Tamales candy, it might be worth retracing your steps to determine if you are really free of your food addictions just yet.

As I alluded to above, the real reason for avoiding the starchy foods on the above list is for weight management. I want you to continue to feel the weight fall off this far into the program. These foods will inhibit that endeavor.

Since we are now talking about weight loss let me mention something else. I considered this quite inspiring as I discovered it about my efforts. The further we get into this way of eating, the more you will clearly see (if you haven't already) that it's hard to eat this way in our modern society. To do this right you could very well begin to be viewed as a fanatic. But that should be perfectly acceptable to you at this point. You should relish working toward becoming a fanatic. A slim, healthy fanatic. This beats the hell out of the alternative—an obese, sickly conformist.

So, let's summarize this chapter a bit. Starches are not bad in the same way that gluten and sugar are bad. They don't represent the same degree of danger. They could be addictive but their effects will not be anything like the addictions suffered through the consumption of gluten and sugar. Many of them will spike blood glucose which leads to food cravings which, worst of all, leads to weight gain.

Bottom line? If you'd like to keep losing weight, add all of the above starches to your excluded list and stay away from them for a full 21 days during this phase. When you're ready to eat them again, test them one at a time and see what they do (or don't do) for you and then decide if you really want to add them back in.

PART IV: OTHER TOXIC CONSUMABLE GOODS

This chapter will be dedicated to defining all of the rest of the stuff that wouldn't be considered paleo-inspired, and therefore ready for admission to your excluded list. It not only includes incompatible foods for your new lifestyle but I have also included some of my own recommendations for adopting other healthy habits related to paleo living outside of just eating better.

In the last chapter we talked about starches and, in case my stance on starches is unclear at this point, let me state that I am not anti-starch whatsoever. In fact, I absolutely love spiralized, sautéed sweet potatoes utilized as a faux pasta to smother with all of my favorite homemade sauces. I eat them quite regularly. My problem with starches (and this should be your problem with them as well) is they can be the culprit in an otherwise clean paleo diet when weight loss stagnates or body mass increases inexplicably. The simple solution for me has always been to lay off the starches for a while until things tighten up a bit. That is my *only* problem with starches (excluding the starches I will be condemning permanently in this chapter). But don't forget that most of the starchy foods listed in the last chapter are not all that nutrient dense. You could live without them altogether if you wanted to.

The overarching theme of this chapter (and also for paleo living in general) is the question of whether or not engineered foods (and other consumable products) can be compared equitably, on the basis of healthfulness for human beings, to what our own Mother Nature is able to provide for us.

The experts appointed to the health of our nation say that scientifically engineered consumables not only line up with what nature can offer but they far surpass such offerings. Just watch any TV commercial trumpeting the praises of a processed food product. Chances are the nutritional benefit of the product will be front and center and likely a main selling point. Listen closely to the implied nutritive superiority of such products over any natural alternative. Why would you eat a dumb old carrot when you could have "Brand Q" (i.e., super-fortified, ridiculously nutritious processed product)? Huh?!

In spite of the numerous leaps in scientific study in this area to date, I (along with the rest of the paleo community) have taken the other side of the debate and feel that processed foods are not superior whatsoever. The sad truth that most consumers are blind to is the fact that such foods are a blatant step *backward* from nature's offerings. And it's not even close. Recall my comparison of reduced fat Oreo's to steamed broccoli from the introduction of this book. It still isn't technologically possible to inject a food item with nutrients and have it compare favorably with a natural food. Naturally-occurring nutrients always have a symbiotic relationship with other compounds present in that food to the degree that most will *require* these other substances in order to be properly absorbed into the body. Without this relationship you simply have a number on an ingredient label which states how much of the injected nutrient will be in your serving of the food but not an accurate reading of how much will actually be able to be utilized within by your body. If you vote for broccoli, then keep reading.

With the only supposed merits of processed foods now being reduced to flavors you can't get from anywhere else and the comfort they provide, I think it is time to start craving something else. It won't be long from this point in the program before your body will start longing for the nutrients found in natural food rather than the chemical agents added to engineered food. This can be to such an extent, the longer you go without processed food, that what used to be *delicious* to you may very well become *disgusting*. Case in point, my past obsession with Ben and Jerry's ice cream. I haven't had this former go-to treat of mine for many years now and couldn't imagine ever eating it again. Back then, I didn't have a particular flavor I was taken with. A pint of any of them would do (oh yeah, a pint was one sitting). The thought of it now turns my stomach. I imagine that, as cleansed as my body has now become of these types of toxic foods, anaphylaxis would likely ensue for me as a result of my ingestion of Ben and Jerry's today.

Honestly, if all you are able to accomplish from reading this book is that you *permanently* eliminate gluten and added sugars from your diet, you will be doing yourself a giant favor. And you will be adding years onto your life in the process. My bet is that won't be enough for you, though. Once the hard work is done (which it mostly is, by the way), you'll be so fired up about feeling good that you won't want to ingest *anything* that could spark an adverse reaction in your body. That's what is spelled out in the rest of this chapter—things that are extremely likely to spark a reaction (that is, a *negative reaction*) in your body. Contrast this with how you were instructed to test foods you are reintroducing. You are mostly looking for *no reaction* (keeping in mind that negative reactions can be disguised by your body) or, better yet, a *positive reaction*. It seems elementary but keep this in mind.

Beyond gluten and added sugar (and starches if you're trying to lose weight), here's my list of items (food or otherwise) that just are not optimal for anyone to consume. They are listed here because they are either capable of causing addiction or other negative reaction or because they are a known carcinogen. All reasons not to give them access to your esophagus anymore. Since you've worked so hard to get here, you are much better off just adding these items to your excluded list and not thinking twice about it. They're bad. Do some research if you're not convinced.

1.) <u>Corn</u>. What is wrong with corn? Let's start with what corn is not. It is commonly believed that corn is a vegetable. Vegetables are good. That is, unless you're trying to lose weight and then you just limit the starchy ones. Well, corn is starchy, but it isn't a vegetable. It is a grain. Grains are bad. All of them. Why are they bad? It actually becomes quite obvious, when the composition of grains is analyzed with some scrutiny, that they were never meant to be eaten by human beings. They really aren't meant to be eaten by *any creature of any kind whatsoever,* to be honest. Grains contain compounds called *lectins* which are also commonly found in most representatives of the plant kingdom. However, grains seem to have these lectins in greater abundance than most other plants eaten by human beings. Lectins are toxic and intended to be. They are a defense mechanism of the plant to ward off any creature who would eat its seed. The problems caused by ingesting lectins are enough deterrent for most animals that they're not interested in most grains at all. Not us humans, though. We love our "healthy whole grains." Intolerance to lectins is believed by many experts to be the *other* reason (aside from reactivity to gluten) why so much of the population reacts adversely to grain consumption. Lectins are not digestible and by being completely indigestible they create a host of problems within the human body. I want to remind you again that this isn't a scientific book. This is a practical book. If you want to know the precise science behind why lectins are bad, it's out there in abundance. Look it up. I will just say that if a skunk wanted to spray me with his defense mechanism, it wouldn't be too long into the process before I got the message and would be running in the other direction. Listen to the plant already. You don't need its seed that badly. Note: There are lots of reports out there that directly contradict the findings that lectins are harmful (I don't put much stock in them). But, I suppose you could do some self-testing here if you felt you needed to. Everybody loves hot buttered corn-on-the-cob at a Summer picnic after all. Is it going to kill you? I hope not.

2.) Rice. Yes, it is a grain. Therefore, everything that applies to corn above applies to rice with one exception. All of the offending toxic matter in rice seems to be concentrated in the bran, or outer layer of the rice grain. So, brown rice (or whole grain rice) is the form of this grain you really want to stay away from because it still has the bran intact. When the bran is removed the result is *white rice*. In reality, when the bran is removed so is any nutritional content that may have also been present before. So if you're OK with a nutritional void that adds a lot of starch to dishes (in other words, spiked blood glucose and the potential for weight gain), go for it. I eat white rice on infrequent occasions, to be truthful. There are worse options for sure.

3.) Legumes. Legumes are beans and they are starchy so they're not good for those trying to get or stay lean. They are also somewhat controversial within the paleo community. And it's not a matter of a lack of nutrition. It's that they might be anti-nutritious. I am referring to the *anti-nutrients* found in legumes (and also in grains). Phytic acid is one of these anti-nutrients and it is the most abundant of them within the legume family. Phytic acid and anti-nutrients in general, as the theory goes, inhibit nutrient absorption within the body effectively rendering the substance they are found in devoid of any nutrition whatsoever. So it's not nutritious, its starchy and it makes you fart.

Why do you want to eat this again? There's a debate that rages with regard to anti-nutrients that is similar to the one concerning lectins so draw your own conclusions. I don't eat legumes anymore. I don't miss them. But, I didn't love them in the first place.

4.) Oils. Wait, what am I going to cook with? Relax, I am not kicking all oils to the curb. Just *industrial seed oils*. Say what? These are commonly referred to as "vegetable oils" but they have little in common with carrots, cauliflower or zucchini as the name would imply. The most common (and most dangerous) of all of these are canola oil, soybean oil, corn oil, peanut oil, cottonseed oil, sunflower oil and safflower oil. The problem is mostly in how they have to be harvested. They can't be simply cold-pressed (which basically means the oil is extracted only through pressure) like some of the truly healthy oils I will talk about in a moment. Instead they must be extracted chemically (with deadly compounds such as hexane) or through the use of extremely high heat. They are then bleached and deodorized with more chemicals. And *then* you get to eat them. Mmmmm mmmm. They are very high in PUFA's (polyunsaturated fatty acids) which makes them very unstable chemically. They can be slightly less toxic unheated but when heat is applied (as in cooking) they become rancid and oxidized (this is bad) and are then a horrible resemblance of something that is supposed to be "heart healthy" as they are so often marketed. Truthfully, most of them are already rancid before they even reach your pantry due to their prior exposure to extreme heat and their own instability. As always, do your own research here. I am not going to say do some self-testing because I don't agree that any of these are OK if you can tolerate them. Wrong. *They are deadly for everyone*. Weird that they have been around for so long now and no one thought twice about them until recently, huh? That kooky government of ours. They're such kidders. As for oils that are good to eat, I would stick to the few I will mention here—coconut oil, avocado oil and ghee. They all have their own positive nutritive value with no drawbacks. Coconut oil is a great choice for cooking as it holds up to very high heat cooking (450-500 degrees F) with no oxidation. There are two types of coconut oil—extra virgin and refined. Extra virgin coconut oil has had the least amount of processing done to it but it smells and tastes like coconut. And it will add this flavor to everything you cook using it. If you can live with that then it should be your first choice. Refined coconut oil is tricky because it *could have* undergone the same chemical bath that industrial seed oils go through. Look for refined coconut oil that clearly states "no chemicals," "no hexane," "cold pressed," "mechanically pressed" or something of this nature on its labeling. If it doesn't say anything to this effect, count on it being chemically extracted. The refined version of coconut oil has no coconut smell or taste whatsoever and, when you find a safe variety of it, has all the same benefits of extra virgin coconut oil. Avocado oil is usually made by pressing only with no chemical treatment, but you'll want to verify this through the labeling on the brand you choose. It also is a very high heat oil (450-500 degrees F) with no real flavor of its own to impact your dishes. Lastly, ghee, which is really just clarified butter (whereby milk solids and water are removed from unsalted butter leaving pure butterfat), has a much higher heat durability (up to 485 degrees F) than the butter it is made from. It is great for sautéing foods and adds a delicious buttery hint to everything. Notice I left off olive oil, the darling of the famous Mediterranean Diet. This is on purpose. OK, I suppose you could have olive oil, but you'll have to be very careful with it. As with all healthy oils, you should settle for pressed varieties exclusively but *you should only ever eat extra virgin olive oil*. Light and extra-light versions are "cut" in order to tame the strong olive flavor of extra virgin olive oil and guess what they're cut with? You guessed it, industrial seed oils. Stay away from these versions of olive oil and be aware that cutting oils are curiously rarely mentioned on their ingredient labels. And never cook with olive oil. It doesn't hold up to high heat at all. But as you would guess, olive oil is great for homemade salad dressings and cold sauces. So enjoy your EVOO in this manner to your heart's delight.

5.) Toothpaste. We have been told for so long that fluoride is one of the remarkable breakthroughs of the century that it is hardly ever questioned. If we don't want to lose our teeth, we need fluoride added to our toothpaste. And just in case that's not enough, let's slip some into our drinking water too while we're at it. And let's not forget the likelihood of getting even more fluoride from the food and drinks we consume that are processed with fluoridated water. I don't want to spend a lot of time with this. My dental health has improved dramatically since I have switched over to a paleo-inspired diet full-time. My teeth are whiter and stronger and my gums are much healthier. The change is strictly diet-related and has nothing whatsoever to do with fluoride. In fact, for the past year I have only brushed with Tom's all-natural toothpaste *without fluoride* and I only drink purified, fluoride-free water because I intentionally want to minimize the risks in case the bad reports about fluoride wind up being the factual reports about fluoride. Studies out there implicate fluoride in maladies from muscle disorders to brain damage. It accumulates in the body, mostly the bones. No thanks. I don't need anything accumulating in my bones without my permission. I can live without fluoride, thank you very much. By the way, fluoride isn't the only toxic agent in most toothpastes. Check the ingredients and do some more research. Why do you think the warning on the label says to not swallow it? Yeah, good luck with not swallowing any.

6.) Teflon. This might wind up being a matter of finding the lesser of all evils when it comes to cookware choices. Teflon, is a brand name for nonstick cookware coated with PTFE (polytetrafluoroethylene). If overheated, PTFE is reported to release fumes which have been shown to cause flu-like symptoms in human beings. Further, polychlorofluorocarbons are released into your food when using these types of pans for cooking. This sounds bad. It likely is if reports claiming such are to be believed. Worst of all, PFOA (perfluorooctanoic acid), a component of PTFE, is a suspected carcinogen. OK so Teflon is obviously bad (as you may have already heard prior to reading this). But it's so convenient! Yep, but so are most of the other options below. Let's look at them closer. Listed in order of their presumed safety priority, the remaining options are ceramic, cast iron, stainless steel and aluminum. Ceramic cookware is considered best because it does not leach any metals into your cooking. It is a super slick surface and has better non-stick qualities than Teflon. This is not to say that there aren't still contrary studies out there about the relative safety of ceramic coatings. Cast iron pans are not non-stick at all until they are seasoned (use a safe high heat healthy oil such as coconut or avocado oil for this). They do leach metal into your food but it is in the form of iron which is considered a healthy and necessary mineral to human physiology. However, some would argue that it leaches *inorganic iron* into our dishes rather than *organic iron* (which our bodies are more readily able to use). They feel that inorganic iron remains in some proportion within the body's tissues if not fully eliminated. These deposits are purported to potentially lead to further health problems. Controversial yes, but still better than the next two options. Stainless steel pots and pans reportedly leach the compounds nickel, chromium and molybdenum into foods cooked in them. Unlike iron, these are not usable by the body at all and therefore it is speculated by many that stainless steel cookware is completely unsafe. Aluminum is the singular toxic element which leaches into cooking with aluminum cookware. Aluminum builds up in body tissues and has links to Alzheimer's disease and other health problems. Aluminum is by far the riskiest of these choices.

7.) <u>Microwaves.</u> Not really food but definitely consumable, microwaves do not need to be part of our diet. Here we go with yet another topic with loads of controversy swirling around it. Invented in 1946 but not really rolled into meaningful production until the mid-50's, the microwave oven is the tool of choice to produce a crispy outer crust on your favorite Hot Pocket variety. But, what can it be used for now that you are ridding your body of toxic consumable products and assimilating into paleo-style eating? Absolutely nothing. Throw it away (unless it's bolted to the wall between the cabinets above your stove). It seems like an oxymoron to say "safe exposure to radiation." Atom bomb fallout is pretty bad I hear. So are x-rays. But you're telling me I can safely stick a frozen block of food into a cold box, press a button and through the magic of electromagnetic radiation that food gets "cooked" from the inside out (in a matter of seconds) while the box never heats up whatsoever? The filling in a Hot Pocket becomes molten food lava yet the inside walls of the box are cool to the touch. Hmmmm, have you never questioned the safety of this process before? No matter, really. Safe or not. You have no use for a microwave oven anymore. Since you prepare your own food now and microwave ovens are reserved for the quick heating of convenience foods or reheating leftovers, the usefulness of this appliance has been depleted for you. As for leftovers, don't be tempted to stick them into the magic box. Heat them up in a pan (preferably ceramic) on the stove or warm them in the oven. One last point, who said microwave ovens are safe anyway? That darn government of ours. Aren't they the ones who still say to eat more whole grains? I rest my case.

8.) <u>Tap water</u>. Heavy metals, human and animal waste, petroleum, pesticides and just about anything else you can think of that could contaminate a water supply are what your municipality has to confront in order to produce "safe" water for you. Do you trust them to do that for you? Studies show they are mostly letting you down. Instead, do some further purification with a filtration system of your own. And make absolute sure your filtration system can eliminate the fluoride our friendly government adds back into the water once they feel it's clean. Your next best choice would be to find a bottled water company with a good reputation for producing water that tests well. Be sure to research this thoroughly.

9.) Artificial sweeteners. I have talked about this topic already to some degree in the previous chapter regarding your addiction to sugar. Consequently, I won't talk much more about it here except to say that we all have heard the warnings about saccharin, sucralose and aspartame (the probable carcinogenic nature of each of them being the most damning). So, since there's been enough said on those already let me just mention the rest of the artificial sweeteners that may also be killing you. Sugar alcohols, which include erythritol, glycerol, lactitol, maltitol, mannitol, sorbitol, xylitol and others, are said to occasionally produce a laxative effect. But in my experience with these (maltitol in particular; not so much with xylitol), this result of consumption was not just a *potential* side effect. It was very real. It was like Ex-lax on steroids but without the gentle warning. To me, that side effect indicates enough of a problem with consuming sugar alcohols that I don't have to revisit the experience ever again to know there's a safety issue here. I will listen to my gut (pun intended) on this one. Other chemical sweeteners you should never put in your mouth are acesulfame potassium (also called acesulfame K, ace K, ACE), alitame, neohesperidin dihydrochalcome (NHDC) and neotame. But, never forget that sucrose (table sugar) is increasingly being implicated as the *most carcinogenic* of all sweeteners (over all chemical sugar substitutes). So far, at this period in human history, it seems that coconut sugar and stevia present the least cancer risk of any of them.

10.) Allergens. Ever heard of FALCPA? This is the FDA's Food Allergen Labeling and Consumer Protection Act of 2004. This act requires the identification of ingredients that belong to (or contain any protein derived from) their list of the eight most common food allergens. These are milk, eggs, fish (e.g., bass, flounder, cod), crustacean shellfish (e.g., crab, lobster, shrimp), tree nuts (e.g., almonds, walnuts, pecans), peanuts, wheat and soybeans. This certainly is not a list of *all* possible food allergens. In fact, it is estimated that the true count of allergenic food ingredients numbers greater than 160 or so. My philosophy, when it comes to food allergens, is *eat what suits you*. You shouldn't feel like crap (or go into anaphylactic shock) after a meal. If you suspect anything of being a problem, use your self-testing tactics. Drop it entirely for 14 days and then try it again and see what happens. With regard to the FDA's list above, I definitely recommend shunning the peanuts and soybeans. They're legumes, remember? You already don't eat wheat. As for the rest of the list items, why not assume that since a pretty good section of the population reacts negatively to them maybe there's a message in there for you? And remember that your body can hide food reactions from you. At the very least, maybe you should eat them in more moderation than other foods just in case.

11.) <u>Chemicals</u>. Do you know what's in your food? This one is simple. Take a look at the ingredient list for a food product. If you can't pronounce it, you probably ought to do some research on it. Most of the really bad things finding their way into processed foods are artificial flavors, artificial colors, sneaky new words for sugar or wheat, flavor enhancing substances or ingredients used to improve texture. Save your health and do an internet search on it before you eat it.

Again, this list is designed to get you thinking about your health in other ways beside just what you eat. Did I cover everything with this list that could cause you problems and shorten your life span? Nah, this list could be a lot longer. We didn't even get to alcohol yet. That gets a chapter of its own.

What else is bad? Smoking is bad. Cell phones are said to be bad. Aluminum foil could be bad and so could a lot of other things. I am not trying to create throngs of paleo paranoiacs with this chapter. I am just pointing out some of the more obvious unhealthy things you may be accustomed to taking into your body in order to get you thinking a little bit. It makes sense to me for you to curb or halt your intake of them because you are treating your body so much better now than ever before. Why not go *all in* and create a complete health plan for yourself that is concerned with *all of the controllable dangers* to your body other than just that which can come directly from what you eat? If I missed a few, take the initiative to add them to your excluded list without my prompting you to.

PART V: A WORD ABOUT ALCOHOL

For some of you, this chapter may be the last straw. You may have stuck with me up to this point but now that I am messing with your booze, you are done with me. If that's you, that's cool. Skip this chapter but keep doing what you're doing from the previous chapters. Lots of paleo people can't quit their booze either but get creative with how to keep calling it "paleo." It's not. Make no mistake.

An occasional drink won't hurt you (we hope) but *alcoholic* cave people just didn't exist in the Paleolithic era of humanity. We don't need the fossil record to tell us this. Cave paintings don't portray a hard day at the office running around chasing gazelle with a crude spear and then unwinding with a few cold ones on the rock sectional in front of a roaring fire. So give it up already. If you can't quit it, that's one thing. But calling it paleo is something you just can't do.

Since you're already pissed off (but strangely still hanging with me), let's talk first about why it's not good for you and then we can get to how you might work alcohol back into your pantry once you have rehabilitated from it. By the way, there are no "good" drinks just some that might kill you more slowly.

In case this chapter gets a little "preachy," just know it is coming from a position of authority. Ask my family and friends and they will tell you that I have been a chronic alcohol abuser right up until a few years ago. This was for a matter of several years lasting into a few decades, to be honest. Some may still only know me as that person, not knowing that I am rehabilitated. I should have enrolled in a 12-step program because I needed it, but I didn't. I was stubborn. I ultimately kicked it on my own (after lots of failed attempts) because I knew it was toxic (and a negative burden on family and friends). I also finally realized that it was pretty asinine that I would eat with such stringent self-imposed regulation yet I could still justify slamming a whole bottle of Cabernet or a six-pack of IPA each night.

But, just because a caveman didn't do it isn't reason enough to rid yourself of it. Remember, I drink coffee and I'm pretty sure that prehistoric Java Man was not named for this delightful hot drink. So, like alcohol, coffee isn't paleo either. In fact, it is probably more likely that a caveman could have stumbled on to fermenting fruit and created a drink from it than it is that he figured out how to roast and grind coffee beans. Regardless, I pretty much use general paleo guidelines as a framework for my diet and fill in the rest with common sense. Forget whether or not it's paleo. When you start looking at alcohol, it is simply downright dangerous for anyone to consume. It is far worse when it is abused.

However, coffee and alcohol are not even on the same playing field. I just used that for illustration. "Six of one, half a dozen of the other," you say? No, you're delusional. You've had enough. Sleep it off. Or drink a cup of coffee.

So why is alcohol so hazardous to one's health?

1.) It is addictive. Wine has lots of sugar in it. Beer is made from grain (as is most hard liquor). But, we're not talking about that kind of addiction (although those substances surely also contribute to the strength of one's addiction to alcohol). We're talking about the overt mind-altering type, like a controlled substance—only this one is legal. This type of addiction is worse than the more passive addictions you have had to food because of the power of the effect. On top of this, it seems to create the illusion that it blocks out the stresses of life for a time while you are in that state. This is why lots of people chronically drink. They aim to recreate this effect time and time again by returning to alcohol. But, guess what? Alcohol doesn't make the stresses of life go away. You always sober up. And the stresses are still there. They will probably eventually need to be dealt with. I learned that they are better dealt with sober rather than plastered.

2.) It whispers in your ear. The mind-altering effect of alcohol usage will reduce you to a hyper-suggestible state. Poor decisions with food choices are an all-too-common result. Poor decisions in other aspects of your life are also possible. It is incredibly easy to develop food addictions while developing an addiction to alcohol. It is also incredibly difficult to rehabilitate from food addictions if you're already an alcoholic.

3.) It will cause excess insulin production and blood sugar spikes. No matter how well you've eaten all day long, if you retire for the evening with a cocktail or two (it doesn't really matter what your drink of choice is), you have basically done yourself more harm than all of the day's food choices combined. I am talking about the chronic drinker here and not someone who can really just sip a half of a glass of wine every now and then. If you have the ambition to lose weight you can kiss success in this endeavor goodbye if you are this type of drinker. It's not going to happen. Even if you literally eat nothing for the entire day.

4.) It is processed in the body differently than other substances. The very minute alcohol enters into the body it is recognized as a poison. For this reason, it gets directly routed to the liver rather than following the normal stages of digestion. This poison immediately gets all of the body's attention and becomes the foremost priority to be metabolized. This is a second reason why it is nearly impossible to lose weight while drinking regularly. Your liver can't help you burn fat if it is consumed with detoxifying you from the poison you just fed it. All of the body's resources get redirected to eliminate the poison while the metabolizing of other food substances present in the body gets placed on indefinite hold until this is accomplished. A healthy body being fed the right foods isn't supposed to operate this way, as you might guess. I found that the fatty layer on my body representing the "last few pounds" that so many dieters struggle with never left me until I gave up alcohol. I got *slimmer* through eating right but I finally got truly lean by also giving up the booze. My liver thanks me to this day.

5.) There are lots of diseases that are unique to alcohol drinkers. This is the unfortunate and underappreciated truth of alcohol abuse. Because most or all of the work to metabolize alcohol is done by the liver, it isn't surprising that most alcohol-related diseases are centered around the pitfalls of an overworked liver. Heavy drinking is about the only way to contract alcoholic hepatitis, fatty liver disease and cirrhosis. It has also been linked to anemia, cancer, cardiovascular disease, gout, dementia, pancreatitis, seizures, high blood pressure and erectile dysfunction. Sudden death from alcohol poisoning is always a real possibility, too. Rather sobering isn't it?

I'm sure you've heard all this before. But, though it may not be just yet, this list may soon become a help rather than a hindrance for you. I know it is a great reminder for me, being sober, when I start to have alcoholic amnesia and crave a drink.

But, here's the million-dollar question for you to ask yourself.

"Can I still be healthy and consume an occasional drink?"

I don't know, can you?

This one is really up to you. Where I am at right now, I can have a half glass of wine and not lapse right back into a bottle a night habit that assumes control of my better judgment. Can you?

If you have an alcohol habit of any kind (and I am assuming you do since you're still reading) you absolutely need to break that habit with a 21-day detoxification from alcohol. Then you can decide where to go from there. Back to abusing it daily is not a good plan. Deciding that it does nothing for you at all and is an expensive habit you can live without is the ideal outcome of your break from it. But make sure you take a break from it. 21 days and no less. Forever is best.

If you still must drink, let's rank your choices from most forgiving to most toxic. Strive for *one drink* on rare occasions. Anything else is asking for trouble.

1.) <u>Wine</u>. Red wine is best. Yes, grapes have tons of sugar, but a good proportion of the sugar in red wine gets transformed into alcohol during the fermentation process. White wines are typically sweeter (with higher sugar content, logically) than red wines. Red wine has resveratrol which has gotten some good press on the nightly news. This doesn't make it healthy.
2.) <u>Vodka</u>. This *only* includes potato vodka. Grain-based types should be avoided like the grain they're based from. Next, you have to ask yourself what am I mixing with the vodka? Most people don't drink it straight.
3.) <u>Tequila</u>. Eat the worm. It's loaded with protein and fits in with the paleo diet much better than the tequila does. Same question on mixers

above applies to tequila if you plan on doing more than just shots with it.

That's it. There's your list if you must have one. If it isn't listed, stay far away.

Beer is made from grain. There are gluten-free beer options but forget them. All beer is fattening as hell and you wind up drinking a whole lot of it to get you where you want to go. Horrible choice.

Whiskey, scotch, bourbon and some gin varieties are all grain-derived as well. They (mostly distillers) say that distillation removes most of the gluten but can we be sure? Um, nope. Move along.

Hard ciders, fruity wines, wine spritzers, wine coolers, sangria and champagne are all sweet. Sweet equals sugar. Sugar equals bad. Skip these too.

SECTION II: NATURAL FOODS – THE GENESIS OF YOUR *APPROVED LIST*

Now we're going to create your approved list. This is the fun part of the program. No more hearing only about what you can't eat. Now it's all about the things you will thrive on. Some of these you may love already but, hopefully, we'll discover some new favorites for you in this section as well. Once your list is fully completed, tear up your excluded list. I'm sure you know what you're not thriving on by now.

It is still amazing to me, two years into changing over to a paleo-inspired lifestyle, how clean the foods I eat now taste. A roasted split chicken breast with the skin left on is greasy. But it's pleasant and satisfying and greasy. I can still remember the contrasting greasy feeling of a large serving of Doritos. It didn't feel that way afterward. It felt revolting quite honestly. And that was back when I liked Doritos.

If Doritos aren't revolting to you yet, they will be. That's if you stay away from them and keep filling up with approved foods from the list we'll create in this section.

Now is a good time to talk about the relationship between macro-nutrients and calories. Macro-nutrients are *protein, fat* and *carbohydrates*. All contemporary diet plans are built on the proposition that weight loss will result if the ideal ratio of each of these macro-nutrients is determined and monitored closely by the dieter. For example, the Atkins Diet plan (depending on which incarnation of it you are drawing from) basically mandates a very low carbohydrate intake, a moderate to high protein intake and moderate to high fat intake. The popular Zone Diet lobbies for a pretty even intake of all three macro-nutrients (40% carb, 30% protein, 30% fat). The near antithesis of the Atkins Diet is the Ornish Diet, an extremely low fat, moderate protein and high carbohydrate mixing of macro-nutrient percentages.

So who is to be believed? Which one works? Really they all (kind of) work.

But, they all demand discipline. And they all promote hunger. And they all require math.

Yuck!

Well, guess what? You're not on a diet. We've had this discussion already. You don't have to worry about what the diet gurus are saying now because you don't need that information. You are eating well and reaping the rewards of it. Nothing any guru can say now will convince you for even a second that you are doing anything except that which is perfectly optimal for your body. You don't count anything, meter anything or limit anything. No portion control or food rationing of any kind needed. Sorry, gurus!

Let's get back to this relationship of macro-nutrients to calories. A calorie is a unit of energy. Calories are most associated with food but the measurement can also be applicable (in some cases) to anything containing energy. At the risk of things getting confusing here and becoming irrelevant to our discussion, we will just stick to how they apply to food. In its most basic sense a calorie is fuel for the human body. Without sufficient calories, our bodies (starting with the vital organs) will eventually begin to fail. This is why diets that are based around rigid caloric deprivation as the sole medium for fat burning can be considered risky. However, you don't see too many of these (calorie-centered) types of diets on the diet scene any longer. It is much more common to see a focus on macro-nutrients. Each of the macro-nutrients can be equated to a caloric measurement as follows:

1 gram of protein = 4 calories
1 gram of carbohydrate = 4 calories
1 gram of fat = 9 calories

Consumable calories do not come from any other source outside of these three macro-nutrients with *the one exception of alcohol*. Alcohol isn't really any one of these macro-nutrients and yet it packs an impressive 7 calories per each 1 gram. Therefore, it isn't necessarily unreasonable to postulate that alcohol must be a macro-nutrient all its own. Food for thought, but it isn't generally recognized as such, however.

Looking at the above table it seems pretty obvious that it would be easiest to limit calories by counting (i.e., *restricting*) fat. Dieters should lose weight so much quicker this way than by counting any other macro-nutrient because the *calories per gram of fat are more than double the calories per gram of either of the other two*. But it isn't really that simple. Nearly all of us have been on a low-fat diet at one time or another in our lives. Yeah, how did that work out for you? I remember feeling starved and miserable. I don't remember much else about it except that I was still overweight when I gave it up.

So why don't diets which severely restrict fat work? As already stated, the body has to have a regular supply of calories (as fuel for energy). When the calories that could have come from fat are eliminated (or, at least, sharply restricted), this creates a situation where calories that fuel the body have to come from somewhere else. These diets rarely turn to protein to make up the deficit because radically high protein diets are considered as dangerous as extreme calorie-restricted diets. You can't really create an excessively high protein ratio with lower ratios of the other two macro-nutrients anyway. This is simply because, no matter how the proportion of macro-nutrients is juggled, protein will always sort of fall in a middling range. You can't really isolate it through food choices, nor would you really want to. Therefore, the bulk of calories in low-fat diets is predominantly sourced from carbohydrates. I think I've made it pretty clear by now that most carbohydrates, such as wheat flour and sugars or starches like corn and alternative flours, cause dangerous blood glucose spikes which result in cravings. The cycle of sugar rush and crash is endless while eating this way and a sense of satiety (or feeling *full and satisfied*) is hard to come by. Even if it is reached it is always fleeting due to the cravings. This would explain why restricting fat and amping up carbohydrate intake repeatedly fails overall as a diet plan. It demands superhuman willpower to restrict one's eating in this way. Most people just aren't that hell-bent when they start such a plan and if they are in the short-term, they don't typically stay that way.

These same principles would also apply to a low-fat, *high-alcohol* diet, if such a plan pops into your head. I tried that one already. No good.

Fat creates a slow expenditure of the calorie energy it contains which creates satiety over the entire process. Think of it as an oak log in a fireplace. It can burn all night. This advantage for the dieter of feeling full for long periods of time is lost when they restrict fat. The depletion of calorie energy from carbohydrates, on the other hand, is much more like a sheet of newspaper soaked in gasoline and thrown into that same fireplace. Poof!! That's about how carbohydrates react in the body. A huge initial expenditure of resources is needed at the ignition stage (insulin production). The burn (sugar rush) is really quick and the recovery stage (crash) can last a few hours. After a nap, you are simply *starving* again.

Still, fat has a bad rep. But blaming fat for our ills isn't as simple as how it was once stated as recently as just a few years ago when fat was considered the enemy of every human heart. To say *fat is bad* just doesn't cut it anymore as a condemnation of fatty foods because we now know that only *bad fat is bad*. Good fat is actually very good (and necessary) for you. It is time you understood this relatively new distinction.

Even our government, who have vilified fat (that is, *animal fat*) for decades, have been compelled to relax their stance a bit lately to recognize the differences in types of fat.

The newly accepted categories of fat include:

Saturated fats (mainly animal products such as milk, butter, cheese and meats; also found in tropical oils such as coconut and palm oils and cocoa butter)
Monounsaturated fats (found in avocados, nuts, olives and some vegetable oils such as canola and peanut oils)
Polyunsaturated fats (mainly vegetable oils such as safflower, sunflower, soybean and corn oils)
Trans fats (usually hydrogenated to increase shelf life)

It's nice that this has been laid out for you. If you do some research on these latest classifications for fat you will find that trans fats are the unanimous new enemy. As such, they are required by law to be identified on the food labels for foods they are found within (they are the only category of fats for which this is so). But, if you keep looking, you might find it interesting that the agencies our government is linked to (like the FDA and AHA) also rank saturated fats as a *very close* second to trans fats in terms of their presumed health risk status. By default, this means that industrial seed oils remain the best types of fats for us to consume. Nothing new here. In spite of these crafty new classifications, this is the exact same thing we've been told ever since they've been telling us such things. Wait, but doesn't the USDA also control most of the country's agriculture (including soy, wheat and corn from which all our vegetable oils come from)? Yeah, that just must be a silly coincidence.

So, whether you realize it or not, you are still being sold on the virtues of vegetable oils and the dangers of animal fats. However, plenty of new (not government funded) research indicates precisely the opposite. Additionally, the size of the authoritative base that still regards this outdated sales pitch as credible scientific data is ever-shrinking. I bet your doctor doesn't believe this anymore. Ask him (or her) about it.

Regardless, let's not get caught up in the controversy. Let's go back to common sense and our previous discussion on *oils* from several chapters ago. Whether you are religious or not. And whether or not you believe in a creator (or at least *causation* of some sort) as a reason why what we know to be actually exists, you have to admit one thing—the earth provides. It is still the only place in the entire universe known to harbor life. So why screw with it? Just give me clean, pressed oils and safe natural animal products. You can keep your bio-engineered seed oils. Forget what category a fat may fall under in the above table, if it follows the template of safe, non-chemical extraction or is naturally-occurring in an animal product, eat it. As far as I'm concerned, anything else is "bad fat" to be avoided. Obviously, our government and I define this differently. But, I recommend that you rely on your own research for determining this for yourself. You should know that at least half of the internet will be opposed to what you're reading here (if not an even *greater* percentage). Take in all the data and use your powers of logic and deduction and form your own opinions.

Speaking of bio-engineering, let's talk about genetically modified organisms (GMO) for a moment. You might have heard of them. This was once a well-meaning undertaking, I imagine.

Why genetically modify a consumable plant or animal species? In the world of agriculture, I see two main reasons. First, by tweaking the genes of certain crops, scientists have actually come up with strains of grain that have become entirely resistant to the pesticides and herbicides that they are continually doused with. These chemical soups kill *everything* but the resistant plant. This means that weeds, rodents and insects don't stand a chance anymore in a field of GMO grain. The second reason to genetically modify crops would be to increase yield. Up to 50% increase in crop yield spells lots of dollars for someone, I'm thinking. But is GMO produce safe? Again, common sense should rule the day here. A better, safer end-product for the consumer should not be confused for the motivating factor behind genetic engineering. It is not. Go back and read this paragraph again and ask yourself if you think that these practices are likely to produce a cleaner, safer product than that of organic practices whereby no genetic tampering is used. Be advised that the licensing of farmers with organic certification has its own problems and controversy surrounding it. And organic does not always mean *pesticide-free*. But, I would still take organic produce over any food which is a known GMO any day of the week.

So, how is bio-engineering conducted on livestock? Well, one practice that is routinely employed is injecting cows with rBGH (recombinant bovine growth hormone), also called rBST (recombinant bovine somatropin). Although, the practice can't really be called genetic modification, this hormone does increase milk production substantially over that of untreated cows. I get that more milk = more dollars, but the unreported part of this equation begs the question of whether or not the practice produces safer (or even, *safe*) milk? Look for "hormone-free," "no rBGH," "no rBST" or "organic" on your milk labels if you are concerned about this (you should be). Another common bio-engineering tactic (but also not genetic tampering) is the administering of antibiotics in animals raised for their meat. So why worry about this? Antibiotics are safe, right? I suppose, but that isn't the issue here. The question is why give an animal an antibiotic in the first place? It comes down to the conditions in which the animal was raised. If I were a farmer concerned only with making a living (and not at all with the welfare of the animals I raise), geometry becomes my friend. Square footage and how many animals I can squeeze into the *fewest* square feet possible becomes my challenge. Here's the problem that creates. When animals aren't able to freely roam about and have to stay cramped in the same quarters day after day, there is no special place for their waste matter to go except down onto the floor below their feet. And then guess where they get to sleep? Living in the same proximity of animal waste matter is not healthy (even for an animal). It leads to disease. Hence, the need for antibiotics. Want to know another reason why all the cows, pigs and chickens are sick in these industrial farms? They eat grain. Grain is bad for people and its equally bad for animals. These cows don't get to eat grass. And these chickens don't get to eat grubs, worms and insects. All they get is grain. Domesticated pigs eat anything. So, it's hard to say what their wild diet would be. But, I want to eat healthy meat, not the meat of sick animals. This is why I look for "pasture-raised" (these could still get grain on occasion) "grass-fed" (probably also got *some* grain) or "free-range" (mostly for poultry products) on the label when shopping for meat products.

These are generalizations and do not represent all industrial farms. Additionally, the rules for labeling and certification in these areas keep changing. But, this is pretty much the way things are as of this writing.

When it comes to animals raised for their meat, you should know that *organic* does not mean pasture-raised, grass-fed or free-range. It only usually means *antibiotic-free* which might suggest a little bit more humane upbringing but that would be about it. And "vegetarian-fed," by the way, is nothing more than a deceitful way to say grain-fed.

If you ever find a package of red meat (beef, bison, lamb, etc.) claiming that it is "grass-finished" then that is the good stuff. This means that the animal subsisted for its *entire life* on nothing but grass. Grass-fed is usually a very misleading label because what it doesn't tell you is the fact that the animal spent the final months of its life moved into a feedlot to eat only grain for the purpose of getting it fattened for slaughter. These animals are referred to as *grain-finished* which just doesn't sound as appealing as grass-fed. It does speak to how fattening grain really is for cows (*and* humans).

Finally, lots of varieties of livestock are given growth hormones in order to get them to slaughter sooner in an effort to maximize profits. Trust me when I say that the meat of animals raised this way looks, smells and tastes abundantly inferior to that of humanely-raised animals fed a natural diet suited for their species. If the lifestyle of the animal shows up noticeably in the quality of their flesh in this way (it does), then it is clearly worth the extra effort (and, sometimes, extra cost) to seek out healthy animal products isn't it? Can't buy in without more proof? Go ahead and do some of your own A/B testing and see for yourself. But be warned that you won't want to go back to factory-farmed animal meats once you do.

Let's get back to our dialogue about macro-nutrients and finish up by talking about how weight loss happens and why understanding this process is important. There seem to be some very rabid misconceptions out there about the mechanics of fat burning so this will be an essential discussion.

It is pretty broadly perceived that the easiest way to lose weight is to cut down on calories. As long as daily calorie intake doesn't exceed daily calorie expenditure, it stands to reason that a person will not gain body weight if this represents a regular pattern of eating for them. True, yet very difficult to quantify as easily as expressed in this way. It just isn't that easy to measure the exact quantity of calories taken in from a meal or snack and it is far more difficult to accurately gauge the quantity of calories burned from the day's activities. People have long believed that the easy way to get rid of the calories from a jelly donut is to hit the gym and work them off through rigorous physical activity. Wrong. Physical activity is a horrible antidote to the damage caused in the body when one chronically spikes their blood glucose through poor food choices. It just doesn't work the way people think it does. You'd need to spend half the day at the gym beating yourself to a pulp to counteract that donut. Typical gym-goers don't generally do that. Additionally, more and more studies are beginning to show that repetitious strenuous exercising can actually be of more detriment than benefit to the human body in the long run. My contention is that the truly easy way to counter the jelly donut is to not consume it in the first place.

My point here is get rid of the calorie counting mentality (if you have one) as you continue forth with this program. It won't work. Just as eating poorly and "fixing it" by working out won't work.

The human body is a machine. There are two types of fuel this machine is able to utilize for proper functioning. One is glucose which is derived from food which is taken in. When more glucose is taken in (or produced) than the body can actually use, much of the excess is stored as *glycogen* in the liver and muscles through a process called glycogenesis. If the liver and muscle tissue cannot accommodate anymore glycogen, then extra glucose is converted into fatty tissue and stored in deposits in various areas throughout the body through a process called lipogenesis.

A human body at rest continues to have an unrelenting need to burn fuel as if it were active. When a person sleeps and is no longer physically feeding themself, they tend to arrive at a metabolic condition known as *ketosis*. Ketosis happens when glucose from ingested food is no longer available in the bloodstream and fuel must be farmed from other sources. This is where stored glycogen and fat begin to get used. When these stores are broken down by the body they convert into *ketones*. Ketones are the body's other form of usable fuel and get burned *only in the absence of glucose*. They are exclusively a *secondary* fuel source. I have essentially just described the fat-burning process within the human body.

So, is there a way we can capitalize on the power of ketosis and *willfully* enter a state of fat-burning instead of sugar-burning? Sounds like you either have to stop eating altogether or become Rip Van Winkle. If you could sleep for a few weeks straight, imagine how slim you might be upon waking. But the truth is you can arrive at a state of ketosis and maintain it through thoughtful consideration of the foods that you eat. Although you can't really feel when your body is burning ketones rather than glucose, there are monitoring devices on the market for those intent enough on knowing for certain. But don't be one of those who get caught up in this. Eating shouldn't be clinical. Once you have a complete approved foods list, you can count on being in a state of nutritional ketosis regularly. The foods on your list will mostly be of the sort that naturally tend to kick start and sustain ketosis.

But what about those who say being in a state of ketosis is a bad thing? Shall we reason through this for them? Carrying around *excess* stored fat, likely gained through poor food choices and nothing else, is the quickest way known to wind up with any of a number of negative metabolic conditions potentially leading to premature death. The *only* way to lose the excesses of stored fat one carries around is through ketosis. So what's the problem? Ketosis is a healthy condition for the body to be in. Carrying extra weight on the body is not.

Let me say one more thing before we finally get to the substance of your approved list. *Planning meal times is a bad idea.*

Huh?

Yes, you heard that right, that is what I said. And, by the way, this is kind of my thinking here. I don't think this concept is broadly considered within the modern paleo community but I am going to use a Paleolithic backdrop for my reasoning.

Once you *really* arrive at paleo-inspired eating (and you are eating exclusively from your approved list) you will understand why I say this. Planning for meals to be eaten at specific times during the day is part of our modern conditioning and does not at all represent how our Paleolithic ancestors might have lived. There was no freezer for storing pterodactyl wings or mastodon steaks. Because of spoilage, meals couldn't possibly have been planned out further than a single day. Hunts could last for days before a kill was made. These realities of early life likely represent the other reason our ancestors would have stayed perpetually slim. Quality of food is only part of it. The *quantity of food* we eat needs to revert to more ancestral proportions as well. Super-size archaeopteryx nuggets just weren't a thing. Of this, I have no doubt.

But let's not get too involved in thinking paleo again. Let's just get our approved list developed and consult that instead. However, I do think we should train our bodies to expect less and demand less. This is a valuable lesson learned from our ancestors who didn't have convenience stores and 24-hour drive-thrus. It is easily achieved when eating properly, so not to worry. It's not a conscious thing you have to prepare for.

The trick is to eat when hungry without exception.

I mentioned this in an earlier chapter. It means you don't stuff the pie hole just because it's 11:30 am and that's when your lunch break is and, dammit, if you don't eat now you won't get a chance to eat again until 6:00 pm.

This is bad reasoning. Very bad.

Once you are adapted to eating this way fully, you won't have false hunger alarms propelled by cravings. Your body will only want food when it starts to feel it should have food. And, as I said before, this can happen infrequently. Far less frequently than when you were listening to your cravings. And when you experience this type of hunger, it's very mild and easy to "turn off" if needed by distracting yourself with other activities. A simple drink of water may accomplish this and keep you from remembering that you're hungry for several hours. This same trick will never work with a mind-altering craving.

Please understand that I am not advocating starving yourself to lose weight. But, the truth is, you may only want to eat once a day. This means you could easily make it until 6:00 pm to eat for the first time in a given day. You don't need to consider this strange or feel guilty about it. You won't die. Quite the contrary. In fact, your body is more than suited to perform this way, so listen to it. The more ketones your body burns, the sharper your mind becomes (according to many new studies on the subject) and the more fat gets burned. Don't worry about getting enough nutrients either. You will be getting far better nutritional value from just one meal of ingredients from your approved list than a whole week's worth of eating your old way would have provided.

Eating can become very social when driven by cultural norms such as "three squares a day." But you should be determined to feed your body properly at the risk of being a social outcast. Your eating style almost demands it. You will raise eyebrows at your 11:30 am lunch break with your bizarre eating (or *not* eating) habits but your outward healthful appearance will justify everything you do. You will make converts who praise you for the brave stand you've taken to defy conventional wisdom.

Or they might call you weird. So what. Be unfazed.

To properly create your approved list, add anything in this section you like. Test out things that are suspect to you or are a known human allergen that you haven't eaten in a while. Remember, don't add beets if you can't stand beets. It's not necessary.

PART I: NUTS AND SEEDS

Don't forget that *peanuts* are not nuts and belong to the legume family. I don't have a part in this section devoted to legumes at all. That is because I don't eat them and neither should you. We talked about why in an earlier section. You won't miss refried beans on your burritos nearly as much as the tortilla they used to be wrapped in. That's because you were addicted to the tortilla. The beans might have also caused cravings. But, now all you get to eat is the meat and the lettuce. Not much of a burrito anymore. And that's good. That burrito was killing you.

Be forewarned that nuts and seeds contain lectins, the same bad guys that are found in grains and legumes. However, lectin activity is not as notably high in nuts and seeds as it is in those other two families. These are a "try them out and see" sort of food category. Some varieties are high in omega-6 fatty acids. This is getting some press lately leading to an outright controversy, so study up on it. Many nuts and seeds can be nasty allergens for some people. But, if they work for you that is great news because they are high in fat. Really high. And this is good fat which will keep you satiated for long periods of time. They are very portable and easy to take with you wherever you go. Popping a few nuts here and there when you might be hungry will go a long way and may just cause you to want to skip a meal (or two). Go with it. Nothing wrong with a handful of pistachios.

That is unless they are packaged with some type of industrial seed oil. This is one of the drawbacks with these handy snack foods. Especially when members of this food family are sold as nut or seed butters. These will almost always will have some type of industrial seed oil in them. So watch out for this. You have been warned.

And keep your nuts and seeds to small servings. They are not the most easily digested food choice you could make which is another reason why I would say they should all be tested.

So should you go with roasted or raw? Salted or unsalted? I don't know. Whatever suits your fancy, I suppose. But, let's take a moment to mention salt. Salt (or, sodium chloride which is the scientific name for table salt) has taken some big hits during the past few decades along the lines of those leveled on saturated fat. Like saturated fat, salt has also seen its status elevated all the way up to *killer*. But, this seems like a pretty severe label to be assigned to a necessary mineral. Yes, a *necessary* mineral. Human beings cannot live without taking in some salt in their diet. However, processed foods contain ridiculously enormous amounts of salt. Knowing this fact about processed foods is what may have prompted our government to warn against adding extra salt to any foods. At least, looking at it *that way* would make some sense as to why it has been recommended for so long to avoid salt like the plague. But when you start eating in the way described in this book, you should never fear the salt shaker again. You will only be getting a fraction of the salt you consumed with your former diet, even if you are a heavy shaker. Say you opt for the salted variety of pistachio nuts, for example, over the unsalted version. Well, an entire cup full would still have far less sodium (320 mg) than a Big Mac (over 1,000 mg). Good thing for your heart that you don't eat those anymore. But, the very least reason for that would be the salt.

I like salt and do add some on occasion to dishes I prepare, but I find the natural flavor of whole foods is so much more enhanced by adding just a hint. I didn't used to feel this way prior to starting this eating plan. Not too many processed foods have "just a hint" of salt. The thought of that is actually laughable. So much so that it should clarify the reasoning behind why getting used to less salt in your meals could take some time. But, once you really get going with this plan, you'll also find that you prefer to tease the palate with subtle saltiness rather than cause your lips to pucker like you just sucked on a sardine.

Here's a list of nuts and seeds you should feel good about eating (unless you find a few that don't agree with you):

Almonds
Brazil Nuts
Cashews
Chestnuts

Filberts (or, Hazelnuts)
Hickory Nuts
Macadamia Nuts
Pecans
Pine Nuts
Pistachios
Poppy Seeds
Pumpkin Seeds
Sesame Seeds
Sunflower Seeds
Walnuts

There are more types of nuts and seeds than this but I have only included the ones you are most likely to find in your grocery or health food store. I haven't tried all of these but I really do love either a handful of pistachios or a spoonful of almond butter as an appetite-suppressing mini meal when I feel just a modest twinge of hunger and where a regular meal would be just too much food. These two choices absolutely excel in this capacity. They are filling and sustaining from the fat content so they will easily derail the hunger you had felt and they will likely keep it at bay for several hours. But anything from the above list will do the same thing. These just happen to be two of my favorites.

You should probably also try roasting chestnuts. They aren't very edible until they are roasted. Very interesting flavor and experience. Heck, you could even try to do it on an open fire as the holiday song mentions. It is easier in an oven, though. This I can tell you from experience.

I am not a big fan of the trendy *superfoods* flax seeds, chia seeds and quinoa (technically, a seed). None of them are nearly nutritious enough to really be considered a superfood for human consumption and they all have lots of detractors who believe they are actually harmful for human health. Do your own research. I never found a good way to eat any of them anyway.

PART II: FRUITS

I hope I haven't appeared to demonize fruits up to this point. It was not intended. I warned in the chapter on breaking your sugar addiction that fruit could play havoc with that undertaking and that fruit juices should be considered just as deadly as sugar. I also recommended that fruit be eaten in moderation if weight loss is a goal. And lastly, I said that alcohol made from fruit isn't a good idea. But that goes for all alcohol, frankly. Other than that fruit is an excellent food choice.

One word of caution, though. If weight maintenance or weight loss are important to you, *dried fruit* will destroy that enterprise quicker than anything else I know of outside of processed crap food. Some thoughts on that:

1.) In addition to the extreme concentration of sugars in dried fruits, more is often added. Huh? Yes, more sugar (or even a sugar alternative) is added to make them taste better. Check your labels.
2.) Portion sizes often become exaggerated. It's easy to eat 6-8 prunes in one sitting but rare that one would do the same with fresh plums.
3.) Sulphur dioxide (a preservative added to most dried fruit). Not really related to weight loss or gain but you might want to research it to see if you want to eat it or not.

Here's a list of common fruits you should be eating. Yes, these are *all* fruits. No vegetables on this list in spite of you wanting to think otherwise.

Apple
Apricot
Asian Pear
Avocado
Banana
Bitter Melon
Blackberries
Blueberries

Boysenberries
Cantaloupe
Casaba Melon
Cherries
Cucumber
Dates (ripe, soft; not dried)
Figs (not dried)
Gooseberries
Grapefruit
Grapes
Honeydew Melon
Horned Melon
Kiwifruit
Kumquat
Lemons
Limes
Loquat
Lychee
Mandarin Oranges
Mangos
Mulberries
Nectarines
Oranges
Papayas
Passion Fruit
Peaches
Pears
Persimmons
Pineapple
Plantains
Plums
Pomegranate
Prickly Pear (Cactus Pear)
Pummelo/Pomelo (Chinese Grapefruit)
Pumpkin
Quince
Raspberries
Squash (Acorn, Banana, Buttercup, Butternut, Summer)
Strawberries

Tangelo
Tangerines
Watermelon
Yellow Squash
Zucchini Squash

What about cranberries? You wouldn't want to eat one without added sugar. Trust me. It's like eating a "crybaby" candy (I still remember those) times ten. No flavor, just tart. No bueno. It can't be on your list because you don't do added sugar. Sorry.

For anything that isn't on this list, like guavas, starfruit or anything else exotic that you might come across, just use your best judgment and then test it out on yourself. If its dried, think twice. If it has added sugar, pass. If it's fresh and raw, go for it.

PART III: VEGETABLES

Alright, now we're going to look at a category where there are practically no disclaimers, provisos or warnings of any kind. Eat as much as you want as often as you want (so long as you're actually hungry). As always, limit the starchy ones (such as sweet potato) if you are concerned with weight management. Eat those with more sugar in them (such as beets) in moderation as well. In Appendix V in the back of this book, these types of vegetables are listed under the heading of "yellow." You'll see what I mean when you get there.

There will be some things that you *think should be on this* list but aren't because they are actually nightshades. Those will be covered in the section following this one.

Artichoke
Asparagus
Beets
Belgian Endive
Bok Choy
Broccoflower
Broccoli
Brussels Sprouts
Cabbage (green and red, Napa or Chinese, Savoy)
Carrots
Cauliflower
Celery
Coconuts
Endive
Escarole
Fennel
Garlic
Green Onions
Greens (Turnip, Beet, Collard, Mustard)
Jerusalem Artichoke
Jicama

Kale
Kohlrabi
Leeks
Lettuce (Boston, Iceberg, Leaf, Romaine)
Mushrooms
Okra
Onion (green, red, Spanish, yellow, white)
Parsnip
Radicchio
Radishes
Rhubarb
Rutabaga
Shallots
Spinach
Sprouts (seed sprouts only; no legumes)
Sweet Potato
Swiss Chard
Turnip
Water Chestnuts
Watercress
Yams
Yucca/Cassava

Make sure that if you are going to eat sprouts that they are *seed sprouts only*, such as broccoli, alfalfa or radish sprouts. If you can't eat the bean, you can't eat its sprout either. This would apply to mung, lentil or other bean sprouts. These are usually found right alongside other vegetable seed sprouts in the produce department of your local store so don't be fooled.

Where are potatoes? As I said, some of the more commonly consumed foods mistaken for vegetables actually belong to the nightshade family. We will look at them next.

PART IV: NIGHTSHADES

Nightshades are a group of plants that belong to the family Solanaceae. The term comes from *solanine* which is a toxic nerve agent that members of this family are known to produce. Belladonna, which is known as the "deadly nightshade" is extremely toxic to human beings and is best known for its appearance in Shakespeare's "Macbeth" being used by the Scottish army to poison the liquor supply of their enemy, the Danes. Nightshades also contain lectins, which we have already discussed ad nauseum in previous chapters.

OK, so yeah, these sound bad. But let's talk about the fact that millions of people eat these foods every day and enjoy them without falling comatose as the Danish army did in Macbeth. Why is this so? Well, like nuts and seeds, the lectin content is low. So there's that. And secondly, the solanine I mentioned earlier is toxic only to *insects that might try to eat the leaves and stems of the plant*. Solanine is not concentrated elsewhere in the plant (such as the flower or fruit), so this really isn't a concern for us. And while belladonna is a nightshade and is incredibly poisonous, other varieties of this family simply are not. However, for those who are sensitive to nightshades, it can feel like you just ate belladonna even though you only ate a tomato.

You can probably guess what I am going to say next. When something such as nightshades can cause problems for a percentage of the human population, it is best to test it out on yourself first before you become convinced it isn't also a problem for you.

Bell Peppers (green, red, orange, yellow)
Eggplant
Goji Berries
Hot Peppers (cayenne, jalapeno, habanero, serrano, chili peppers, paprika)
Pimentos
Potatoes (red, white, yellow, Yukon Gold, Russet)
Tomatillos

Tomatoes

All I can say is it would really suck for me to be intolerant to nightshades. Bacon-wrapped jalapeno poppers are a hands-down favorite food of mine. I'm really glad I can eat nightshades without problems. I hope you will be able to also.

PART V: DAIRY (AND FERMENTED DAIRY)

Right off the bat, let me just say that everything in this section should be tested for your own personal compatibility with it. Some paleo divisions don't recognize dairy at all because of the problems it causes for so many people (it is a very real allergen for some). Where they would say it absolutely wasn't, I say it *could have been* paleo. A caveman might have been able to milk a yak or a reindeer if he really wanted to. That's close enough to a domesticated cow for me. Bottom line is, if you have no problem with it, don't hesitate to eat dairy (and fermented dairy) products. It represents a natural and nutritious family of food products but moderation is probably a good idea regardless.

Dairy Products:
Cream
Half and Half
Milk

Fermented Dairy Products:
Cheeses
Kefir
Sour Cream
Yogurt

Remember that it is not healthier to consume low-fat dairy products over full-fat ones. In fact, it is the opposite. Added sugar is not healthy and it is *always* included whenever fat is removed.

When dairy is fermented, much of the natural sugar present in the milk gets fermented out of it. This makes fermented dairy products preferable over those which aren't fermented (excepting full-fat cream, which is naturally very low in sugar). Whole milk can actually be very high in sugar content so go easy with it.

Raw milk is a whole other argument (as well as a movement, of sorts these days). This is milk which has not been pasteurized (heat-sanitized) but good luck finding any if you don't have access to a rural farm source. Milk on grocery store shelves is highly regulated and raw milk is even illegal to be sold in some states. You won't find any there to be sure. Some health food markets are beginning to carry it but raw milk isn't without its own enduring controversy. This is because heat pasteurization is heralded as a scientific breakthrough nearly along the lines of the discovery of penicillin. The process is said to make milk safer by destroying food borne bacteria that would otherwise present a significant health risk.

So why even risk one's health by drinking milk that *hasn't* been pasteurized?

By the way, I am simply presenting the argument here without taking a side. Don't shoot the messenger.

There are several reasons that raw milk is making a comeback. Trace raw milk back to a farm and you will always find a humane place where cows graze freely and eat grass. There will be no pathetic grain-fed animals in cramped quarters sleeping in feces. So there's that obvious *potential* health benefit over industrial milk. It's healthy milk vs sick milk. And, by the way, this is essentially the same debate as that regarding the health of the *meat* of cattle that rages between grass-fed beef proponents and the other side which supports penned, inhumanely treated, grain-fed animals. There's also the question of whether or not heat sanitizing also renders the nutritive value of the milk void as it destroys bacterial elements. And finally, the deal sweetener for most who have converted to the raw milk movement is their claim that it simply tastes superior and has better texture in the mouth than factory milk.

Again, I'm not much of a milk drinker so I can't offer an opinion either way. I do, however, prefer to purchase grass-fed cheese wherever I can find it.

Pasteurization does offer some extended shelf-life, so raw milk cannot be kept as long as its counterpart.

In limited independent testing (discounting results offered by the FDA and CDC due to probable bias), raw milk has been found to be only slightly more likely to harbor an increase, on average, in bacterial contaminants than that found in pasteurized milk. And those bacteria found are not of the sort that would cause debilitating illness (requiring hospitalization) but only mild gastric reaction. This seems to be a trade-off that raw milk advocates can live with. They're not buying these findings for the most part anyway. The CDC openly admits that their grim findings apply to "improperly handled" raw milk. Makes you wonder whether or not they did any testing at all on "properly handled" raw milk, doesn't it?

PART VI: FERMENTED FOODS

Fermented foods became a game-changer for me when I converted over to this way of eating. I always thought a pickle was a pickle and that refrigerated pickles tasted (and looked) better than the yellowish ones sitting on the shelf for God knows how long. That was the extent of my knowledge on the topic. Boy, did I have a lot to learn.

Now that I have actually entered into the fray of making my own pickles, I find I was right about the refrigerated (minimally-preserved) varieties. When the focus is on freshness over shelf-life, the end product shines a lot brighter. I have developed a much a greater appreciation for this underrated food family than what I had a few years ago. They will be a game-changer for you as well.

Who knew how healthy they were? I sure didn't. Forget store bought probiotic supplements which seem to be so trendy for overall health all of a sudden. Eat a pickle instead. Or kimchi. Or drink some kombucha. Get your probiotics straight from their natural source. That's got to be a better option than taking a pill.

So what makes food that sits around and basically transforms into another kind of food so healthy?

Fermenting is accomplished through the breaking down of carbohydrates (mostly sugars) and proteins by microorganisms such as bacteria, yeast and molds. These types of foods are considered probiotics due to the overall effect in promoting healthy intestinal bacteria (which aids in digestion) and supporting a healthy immune system within the body.

Lacto-fermenting is a process by which a bacteria called Lactobacillus converts sugars into lactic acid. The production of Lactobacillus is typically facilitated through brining, or the addition of the acting agent of salt (in the form of a salt solution) to a food. This is the kind of fermenting I recommend most. And, although it is a simple concept it can produce varied results. I have made good batches and I have produced some pretty challenged batches. They were always edible but the appearance or the mouth-feel of the final product sometimes suffered. This is because proper fermenting of foods is more art than science. But a proper lacto-fermented pickle is the greatest pickle you've ever eaten. This I promise. But it won't compare to what you commonly think of as a "pickle."

For me, a pickle was always that semi-soft, semi-crunchy yellow cucumber (or white one, if it was of the refrigerated variety) swimming in vinegar. In my ignorance, I blissfully enjoyed them thinking I was eating a fermented food. The truth is, these types of pickles are *pickled food*. There is quite a difference.

The reason for the yellowish appearance of pickled food on your store shelves is due to the fact that they (just like the milk from factory farms) are subjected to heat pasteurization. This is so they can last indefinitely in sealed jars on unrefrigerated shelves of grocery stores. This is an obvious benefit for the food manufacturer. The reason they are soaked in vinegar rather than being lacto-fermented in a brine solution is because the vinegar halts the growth of any bacteria that could cause fermentation. This leads to even longer shelf life for the pickled product. And then preservatives such as sodium benzoate or EDTA may also be added to basically create an indestructible food that can be stored in anticipation of an apocalypse. These are commercial pickles. And if you must eat them, I recommend the refrigerated variety because at least they haven't been pasteurized. But they are a far cry from a healthy pickle.

Being that I now have a pretty good grasp on what I am doing when it comes to fermenting foods, I am having a lot of fun with it. I am not an expert on the subject and I am certainly not yet an *artist*. Therefore, I would not have you look to me as an authority on fermentation. There are lots of good books out there on how to do it right. So consult them instead.

Here's a list of healthy fermented foods. Again, this list of foods assumes you have made them yourself and are not eating commercially pickled or prepared foods. Those are not in the same category as what you can produce yourself. The commercial ones may or may not be healthy. But, take great care in what you are doing. There are some costly and potentially dangerous mistakes that can be made by the uninitiated when fermenting foods. The formation of toxic molds is always a possibility as are a number of other potential hazards. So do your homework.

Lacto-Fermented Foods:
Cheese
Cucumber (we are talking about a proper lacto-fermented pickle here)
Kimchi
Sauerkraut
Vegetables (almost anything you can think of)
Yogurt

Mixed Ferments—yeast, bacteria or other:
Kefir
Kombucha
Water Kefir

Mold Fermented Foods:
Bleu Cheese
Brie Cheese
Camembert Cheese
Gorgonzola Cheese
Roquefort Cheese
Stilton Cheese

By itself, yeast presents another way to ferment foods, but its most common by-products of beer, wine and bread have already been excluded for you so there's really no need to talk about that process.

PART VII: FISH AND SEAFOOD

So this category has some controversy surrounding it and lots of these foods are known to be allergens for some people. All I can say is wade into these waters at your own risk.

I love fish. All kinds. I have never found a variety I am not able to eat and fully enjoy without side effects of any kind. The one exception to this is canned tuna. No side effects for me; I just can't stand it. But this doesn't represent a very *natural* state in which to find a fish. And it certainly isn't the paleo way to eat it. Therefore, I can easily snub my nose at this version of fish and stick only to fresh fish (or as *fresh* as I can get it in the Arizona desert). I have no problems whatsoever with shellfish either. I don't love oysters or clams but that is a personal choice and is not based on intolerance of any sort. I say, if you're like me, you should enjoy all the fish and seafood you like. Unless you're concerned about *mercury*.

According to the National Wildlife Foundation, the toxic metal mercury can "adversely alter the neurological and reproductive systems of humans and wildlife." It is believed by certain researchers that the mercury content present in the flesh of certain seafood varieties can accumulate in the tissues of those who eat it. I make no recommendation for you either way here. Call me a hypocrite if you will for not using Teflon and eating swordfish. I am taking the natural product over the man-made one and hoping for the best. In my defense, I have read every report I can get my hands on regarding this debate and am not yet convinced of there being enough of a problem to give up seafood. For every article in support of the toxicity of fish I find two more debunking the claim. I can't say the same about reports on the dangers of Teflon.

Yet the tests in the area of seafood toxicity continue, so definitive answers may be forthcoming. I am willing to give it up if an undeniable study emerges (or if I keel over from mercury poisoning). Like myself, you should stay tuned.

One thing you might want to pay some attention to, if you do decide for yourself that eating seafood is acceptable for you, is the subject of *farm-raised* vs *wild-caught*.

"Oh wow, one more thing to look for on a food label!"

"When will it end already?!"

Soon enough, I promise. Almost there.

The debate between farm-raised and wild-caught seafood comes down to a simple principle—mass production. Why spend days at sea trying to harvest cod or sea bass in treacherous waters when you could just raise thousands upon thousands on a fish farm?

I urge you to do your own research here at the risk of my steering you in one direction over another. But suffice it to say that conditions in a fish farm tend to be similar to those in a commercial livestock farm. Very unnatural. And these fish tend to have concentrations of antibiotics and pesticides in them. You can guess why the antibiotics are used based on our previous discussion on the subject. The pesticides are typically used to fight sea lice or other parasites. Obviously, these same substances would not be found in wild-caught seafood.

Atlantic salmon, catfish, tilapia, seabass, cod, shrimp and scallops are some the types of seafood in your grocery store's meat department that are likely to be farm-raised. These are all pretty disgusting choices in lieu of wild caught alternatives, in my opinion. But make sure you form your own opinion instead, based on your own research.

Seafood labeled as *organic* will always be farm-raised so that will be of no help to you in the decision-making process.

Here are your typical (and a few not-so-typical) options for fish and seafood at your local grocery chain. Not all of these are ocean fish; there are a few freshwater types thrown in that you might also find in your meat department.

Abalone
Amberjack
Anchovy
Atlantic Cod
Atlantic Salmon
Basa/Swai
Bass
Black Sea Bass
Catfish
Chilean Sea Bass
Clams
Cockle
Crab (King, Dungeness, Snow)
Crawfish/Crayfish
Flounder
Grouper
Haddock
Halibut
Lobster (Spiny, Norway, Rock)
Mackerel
Mahi-Mahi
Monkfish
Mullet
Mussels
Ocean Perch
Octopus
Oysters
Pacific Cod
Pike
Pollock
Rockfish
Salmon (Chinook, King, Sockeye, Alaskan, Pink, Coho)
Sardines
Scallops
Sea Bass (European)
Sea Urchin
Shad
Shark

Shrimp/Prawns
Smelt
Snapper
Sole
Squid (Calamari)
Sturgeon
Sunfish
Tilapia
Trout
Tuna
Whiting

There's also a whole other list you could create of fresh-caught freshwater varieties of fish (such as perch, bluegill, rainbow trout, walleye, etc.) if you happen to be an inland fishing enthusiast. Provided they are coming from safe waters, these should be much better options than any you could find from the above list. And catching your own ocean fish would always be preferable to commercial offerings as well, but who does that? I live in the desert.

Check the ingredient lists for smoked and preserved (canned) fish for any ingredients that wouldn't be otherwise permitted on this eating plan. There is a pretty extensive discussion on cured/uncured meats in the chapter on pork coming up.

One final consideration to ponder is where your seafood is from. In other words, from which country was it imported? Very little of the seafood in our grocery stores is domestically caught (or raised). Of this mass of imported fish, only 2% or so are inspected for contaminants before being shipped to your grocery store. Additionally, some countries have had a worse reputation at times than others when it comes to providing quality seafood. Check your headlines to see who is in the news on this front at the moment.

Moral of this chapter? Be way more diligent in the selection of the seafood you eat than you have been.

PART VIII: POULTRY AND AVIAN GAME MEATS

Chicken usually comes to mind when one hears the word *poultry*, but the term covers a lot more ground than that. Turkey is poultry. Bet you didn't know that. So is duck, goose and any other domestic fowl. Wild birds don't qualify.

Vegetarian-fed or *vegetarian diet* are not really a desirable thing to be looking for when shopping for poultry (even though it will be proudly plastered all over the packaging) as it simply means grain-fed. *Free range* could mean that the birds were able to get a little more variety in their diet but were probably fed grain as well. At least, they were happier.

Try to always buy *organic* when shopping for poultry. This actually means something here, unlike using the word to describe fish.

And try to never settle for pre-cooked (rotisserie) whole chicken fryers from your grocery store if you can possibly help it. These were some of the sickest, most pathetic birds known to man prior to winding up under that heat lamp. It's not that hard to roast a whole chicken. Set it and forget it. And it will taste much better (that is, if you get a healthy bird). The *convenience* of the pre-cooked whole chicken isn't worth the trade-off. Just saying.

The nutrient composition is different from white meat to dark meat in poultry. I wouldn't say one is preferable over the other because both are great food choices. White meat has about half the saturated fat of dark meat. This is why it has always been pushed as the healthiest part of the chicken. But I'm here to tell you that a boneless, skinless chicken breast is not the healthiest way to eat chicken. As I mentioned in the introduction to this section, it is now known (except by our government who has an agenda for staying oblivious) that saturated fat is not bad fat at all. It is really a good fat we should eat regularly. Therefore, embrace the leg and the thigh and, for goodness sake, leave the skin on the chicken breast. It's the best part.

Meat cooked with the bone intact is always superior in flavor to meat separated from all bones before cooking. So get inspired to roast split chicken breasts (with the skin left on, of course), or even a whole fryer. You'll be missing out on a whole new world of flavor (and healthy fat) if you stick to your tired old boneless, skinless breasts.

Some of the birds listed below are game birds and will not ever be seen in your grocery store's meat department. They must be hunted and killed to be tasted. Not for me. I'm good with grocery store free range chickens, thanks.

Chicken
Cornish Hen/Cornish Game Hen
Duck
Goose
Guineafowl
Pheasant
Quail
Squab
Turkey
Wild Turkey

Watch ingredients in preserved versions (canned, sausages, liver products, etc.) of the above.

Brining (in salt solution) is a recent discovery of mine and a fantastic way to prepare poultry for cooking. You'll never suffer with dry meat again if you brine first. And the end flavor will be unmatched. Your house guests will marvel at your ability to cook. I have done a whole turkey this way all the way down to split chicken breasts. Even when chicken is diced and added to recipes, as in stir-fry recipes, brine it first. It's worth the extra effort. It's very simple to accomplish and it would seem like it could work for all birds. But don't quote me on that. Look it up.

I know I talked a lot about chicken and not much else in this chapter. That's because, from that list above, I am an authority on chicken and not much else. I smoked a turkey for Thanksgiving this year (after brining for 2 full days) and it was absolutely the tastiest turkey I've ever eaten. But, beyond that, I can't speak from experience about any of the other birds on the list. Sorry.

PART IX: PORK AND WILD BOAR

I am sorry to say that this is another food category in which I don't have extensive experience. For a few decades I never ate pork in any form, thinking I didn't care for it. *Oops!* Turns out I *do* care for it. Quite a bit. In nearly all its forms. And when my food choices diminished while I was transitioning over to the way I eat now, it became a big player. Therefore, I will do my very best to enlighten you on the merits of this food category in spite of my limited exposure to it thus far.

Bacon is yummy.

Who knew? For the longest time, I didn't.

Is it diet food? Turns out it performs pretty well in such a capacity.

If you can't yet wrap your mind around the reality that bacon might actually be (*gasp*) *healthy*, maybe some outside research on the subject is warranted. But before you head there, let me just say that the two most damning elements of bacon have always been the salt and the fat. (So what's the problem again?) It isn't trans-fat that is found in bacon. It's good old *heart-healthy* (yeah, I said it) saturated fat. Consequently, bacon excels as a diet food because the fat will keep you satiated for hours on end. And we already talked about the need for sodium in the diet and the fact that you will be getting so much less in your diet now that you are eating according to this plan. Bacon will be a big help in making sure you get enough. Get rid of what remains of your notion that bacon is the food of obese heart attack victims. That is the result of brain-washing with bad or manipulated data. It isn't remotely true.

Who hates bacon the most? Our government—the ones who sold us this bad data from the start. Well, who cares? You don't listen to their biased opinions anymore when it comes to food choices. If you decide to do further research on bacon because you're not yet convinced, make sure that you are looking at current data and not outdated findings. And check that it isn't presented by any agencies that could be backed by our government.

Let's talk about how you are going to want to go about reading labels when it comes to pork products. Keep in mind that this applies only to prepackaged preserved foods in this category. Fresh pork meats will not have such labels.

There is a big distinction to be made between the age-old curing process of meats in general and contemporary *cured* (and *uncured*) meat products. For centuries, the only way to cure (preserve) meats was to salt them liberally or smoke them. Sugar (or honey) was regularly added to salt cures to lessen the harshness of the salt. In the wake of progress, however, new methods have emerged. But, I hesitate to call this change *progress* and tend to prefer the old ways.

The change I am talking about is in the use of nitrate and nitrite curing salts (these are sodium nitrate and sodium nitrite, also called *nitrates* and *nitrites*). Sodium nitrite is a chemical derivative of sodium nitrate, a naturally occurring substance. The difference between cured and uncured when it comes (mostly) to pork products lies in the usage of these salts. Any pork product labeled as *cured* will have utilized one or the other (or both) of them isolated as a primary preservative and any labeled *uncured* will not. I have my own opinion here (as usual) and I caution you that this is yet another controversial topic. For my sake, if I eat packaged preserved meats (pork or otherwise), I always verify that it is uncured prior to purchasing. This is a force of habit for me but may be founded on my own unreasonable paranoia as you may determine for yourself by reading on.

Here's the deal with nitrates and nitrites. They add a nice color to the meats they are added to, turning them a natural looking pink or red. But, they also can both convert to *nitrosamines*, a highly carcinogenic agent. Nitrosamines are also commonly found in beer (yet another reason to stay away). Nevertheless, an argument in defense of nitrates and nitrites which is often heard is that some vegetables (such as spinach and celery) also contain them and that they appear in far greater quantity in these natural foods than that which would be taken in by eating processed cured meats. Let's look at this charge a little closer. It is true that certain vegetables contain sodium nitrate, some of which becomes sodium nitrite when eaten (through contact with saliva). Sodium nitrite can form nitrosamines. *But, the vegetables in which sodium nitrate is found all contain antioxidants* (and especially vitamin C) which inhibit the formation of nitrosamines. This is the simple reason why nitrates and nitrites are considered dangerous in cured bacon (or other *cured* meat products treated with them) but not in carrots.

Uncured pork products are on the rise with the recent public awareness of the supposed dangers of meats cured with nitrates and nitrites. Two years ago, I couldn't find uncured bacon. Now my nearest grocery store sells it. Packaging on preserved pork products regularly seems to state "cured" or "uncured." Other meats aren't as consistent in their labeling. Packaged corned beef is a good example of this. You will have to look at the ingredient lists for these other meats to see if nitrates or nitrites are added.

The growing concern over the commercial use of nitrates/nitrites has prompted some regulation by the USDA whereby ascorbic acid (vitamin C) or erythorbic acid (*isoascorbic* acid; derived from vitamin C) is required to be added as an ingredient in cured meats to counter the potential for the development of nitrosamines.

Personally, I question whether this artificial pairing of components seen to work together when occurring naturally in vegetables would be as effective in cured meats. Seems easy enough to just insist on eating uncured meat products and thereby avoid all risk altogether, right?

Well, there's one more part to this whole controversy. The little-known reality is that uncured meat *still contains nitrates and/or nitrites* in spite of the way things are labeled. Say what? Yes, this is true. They are treated with *natural* nitrates from the likes of celery juice powder, beet juice powder, carrot juice concentrate or sea salt (yep, a potential source of them as well). Again, vegetables are a huge source of nitrates so concentrating them into a usable form (liquid or powder) for the function of capitalizing on their nitrate content for curing makes a whole lot of sense. But have we really accomplished anything in making the curing process any safer by doing this? And the whole argument seems redundantly circular if we truly believe that we can avoid nitrates/nitrites by simply curing with salt. Sea salt is also said to contain them. And why wouldn't any other type of sea salt derivative—table salt included—since all our salt comes from a body of salt water in some form?

There you go. I didn't clear up anything for you whatsoever did I? If you're concerned, I recommend that you stay tuned in to the ongoing debate. I have stated that I remain in favor of uncured products, hoping that natural sources for my nitrates/nitrites offer some further protection. But, my bottom line is I will eat these types of foods *infrequently* until this whole mess is resolved once and for all. When I do eat them, I prefer to prepare them myself with good old-fashioned salt. I trust, that when the smoke clears, salt will be exonerated.

Here's my pork list. I mentioned wild boar in the title of this chapter but I am rather ignorant with regard to it. I know some people eat wild boar but I am not much of a hunter. Outside of the Discovery Channel, I have never even seen one to be honest. But, like its cousin the pig, it is super nutritious and fully approved for your purposes here if you happen to have access to it.

Preserved Pork Products (check these closely for other added ingredients that don't comply with this eating plan such as added sugars, industrial seed oils, etc; *cured* or *uncured* is up to you):
Bacon
Canadian Bacon
Capicola
Coppa
Culatello
Ham
Hot Dogs/Frankfurters
Mortadella
Pancetta
Pepperoni
Porchetta
Prosciutto
Salami/Salame/Salumi (Hard, Genoa, Soppressata, Peppered, Cotto)

Sausages (Bratwurst, Italian, Breakfast, Chorizo, Andouille)
Summer Sausage/Kielbasa

Fresh Pork Cuts:
Back Ribs
Belly
Blade Steak
Boneless Loin/Loin Roast
Chops (Shoulder, Sirloin, Boneless, Loin Chop, Rib Chop)
Country-Style Ribs
Crown Roast
Ground Pork
Rib Roast/Rack of Pork
Shoulder/Boston Butt
Spareribs
Tenderloin

Cook these fresh cuts with bones in whenever possible for improved flavor.

PART X: RED MEATS—BEEF, BISON/BUFFALO, VEAL, VENISON, LAMB AND ELK

In the interest of full disclosure, I will say upfront that I have only ever eaten beef, bison (or was it buffalo?) and elk from the meats listed in the title of this chapter. Lambs are cute as hell and veal just breaks my heart. Adorable and/or baby animals are something I just can't see myself eating no matter how hungry I get. This also goes for rabbits and squirrels and lots of small game animals that I'm not even going to mention anywhere else in this book except right here. Pretty prejudiced towards not-so-attractive animals, I know. Sucks for them. I tell myself that cows aren't cute. Why that helps me to be able to eat them I have no clue. But, it wasn't me who made them ugly (*and* delicious).

You've already read that I am not a hunter. So, the flavor of venison escapes me as well.

I think I could eat a wide variety of (ugly) living things; I just can't kill anything. I honestly have trouble killing venomous spiders and the really creepy scorpions native to my Arizona home. I typically trap them and escort them outside rather than kill them.

So there's my quandary.

I'm a full-fledged carnivore incapable of killing my prey.

Things might be different for me if there suddenly wasn't a grocery store meat department nearby and I started feeling a little hungry. I'd have no choice but to sharpen my spear. But, for now it seems like I'm safe shopping there and not refining my spear-chucking skills. At least until the zombie apocalypse comes and the store gets looted and ransacked and all the meat is suddenly gone.

My ethical stance in all of this is I try very hard to ensure that all the animals I eat were treated as well as possible. If the whole world suddenly declared they would only eat grass-finished, organic beef (and other meats), then the industrial animal mills of the world would have no choice but to adapt. Not likely, but I sleep a little better at night doing my small part.

I am a big advocate of eating the whole animal. "Nose-to-tail" is the proper verbiage for this. My problem is I haven't developed a taste for very many of the other parts yet. I will get there (I am hoping), but right now I need to rely on those other markets who are accustomed to (and *prefer*) tongue over chuck roast to make sure no part of the animal, that had to give up their life for our sustenance, is wasted. For now, I will take care of the chuck roast end of things.

Speaking of chuck roast, below is a list of red meats that can be added to your approved list.

Preserved Red Meats (extremely difficult to find any of these that would adhere to the other criteria of this eating plan due to added ingredients such as sugars, corn syrup, soy sauce/soy protein, industrial seed oils or wheat so be diligent in scrutinizing them; nitrates/nitrites also likely):
Beef/Game Sausages or Hot Dogs
Canned Meats
Corned Beef
Jerky/Processed and Formed Meat Snacks/Dried Meats
Luncheon Meats

Fresh Red Meat Cuts (these can be beef, bison/buffalo, elk or game varieties):
Back Ribs
Brisket
Chuck Roast
Filet Mignon
Flank Steak
Flat Iron
Ground Meat
Organ Meats/Offal
Rib Roast
Ribeye Steak

Sirloin Steak
Skirt Steak
Strip Steak
T-Bone Steak
Tenderloin Roast
Top Round Roast
Tri-Tip Roast

Cooking with bones in to enhance flavor is especially noticeable with red meats. Take advantage of the practice whenever possible.

PART XI: WATER

Is this chapter really necessary? Yes.

Do I need to tell you that water is healthy? I would hope not, but that isn't what this chapter is really about.

The reason it is here is because you may not have realized that water is all I have left for you to drink (well, besides coffee). And, that is not a bad thing. Once your addictions are broken, you begin to realize that water tastes pretty darn good. If you really believe it has no taste, it's probably because you still miss soft drinks.

I also have some other things to say about water.

For something as life-giving and necessary as it is to the human species, it's crazy how many people live their day to day lives in a constant state of water deficit. Dehydration is a bad way to die and, yet most people are halfway there most of the time. Part of the reason for this is not because they aren't taking in enough liquids. Most drink whenever they feel thirsty. And many more drink *a lot* of liquid when they do drink something. It's nuts to me that a 32-ounce cup filled up at a convenience store soda fountain only represents a "medium" drink these days. However, the reason they stay dehydrated is *because the liquids they drink are not water*. Gatorade is not better for your body than water. And let's be clear, the only thing in the Gatorade that your body even wants is the water in it. No matter how thirsty you are.

It is estimated that a person can only live 3-4 days without water. To me, that makes water the hands-down most important thing that you should be concerned about getting enough of for your body. Forget about nutrient ratios. That is all taken care of now by your approved list. What isn't covered is how much water to take in and what the quality of that water should be. Well, first of all, in speaking about the quality of the water that you should drink, I really don't think skimping on the price required to get high-quality purified drinking water for yourself (and your family) is a wise idea. The tap water from your faucet isn't a free source of water—you pay a monthly water bill for the service of delivering it to your home. And, it's disgusting. I would never give my dogs tap water to drink. They, like the rest of my family, get a home-filtered version of it designed to eliminate the fluoride and chlorine (disinfectant) that are added to my municipality's water source in order to make it "safe" to drink. So, you're paying for it but, it's dangerous. Spend a little more money and transform that tap into a trusted source of nourishing water. Do your research and a find a filter that can absolutely deliver the cleanest version of this most vital element to your existence. There is a lot more in my city's water that I want eliminated from it including a high enough ratio of calcium, magnesium and manganese to earn it a label of "hard water." While these minerals aren't harmful to drink, they make bathing (and washing a car) annoying. It isn't really soap scum you see in a ring around your tub when hard water is present, it's *mineral scum*, which sounds better but is every bit as difficult to clean.

Here's something else you might not have thought of. You've purchased a filtration system for your tap that engages when you'd like clean drinking water and can be disengaged when using it for any other purpose. So, how about washing dishes? Is there also a filter placed before your dishwasher when traced to your water's source? There should be. That water is bathing the silverware that goes into your mouth. You really don't think that unfiltered municipal water rinses clean do you?

Filters of any kind don't last indefinitely. Change them according to the frequency recommended by the manufacturer.

What about the water you boil vegetables in? Filtered? And, it isn't any safer to steam vegetables instead if you're still using tap water.

How about coffee? Sure, coffee disguises the awful taste of tap water but it hasn't done anything to clean it up. Heating it doesn't kill anything—not to the puny temperature you've heated it to. You need to go much hotter for that purpose. And, even if heating it might kill some bacteria, it does nothing to rid your water of the toxic chemicals added to it. Use purified water in every drink you mix with it.

How much water should I drink? Well, that's a good question. And here's the easy answer. More than you think you should. There's water in a lot of the food we eat so your body does get some from it. But, you are now probably eating a lot less than maybe you ever have in your entire life, so that's not much of a help. And, remember if you had endless amounts of food but no water, you're still dead in 3-4 days. Drink water when you feel thirsty and then drink more at other times. Make sure you drink water when you don't feel thirsty, because guess what? A healthy individual can't really overdo it.

"But, it makes me pee when I drink a lot of it."

Uh, huh. Good job. You're doing it right.

Now, I do need to say one thing about overdoing it. There is a condition called *overhydration* which can affect those with an inclination to retain water. These are persons with diagnoses such as liver disease, kidney problems, congestive heart failure or anyone else with a propensity for water retention. If this is you, check with your physician or other care provider before starting my recommendation to drink more water than you have been. Overhydration affects the proportion of water to sodium in the body creating a severe dilution of sodium which can lead to death.

Speaking of death, let me mention alcohol dehydration. If you drink alcohol, I bet you know what I'm talking about here. If my chapter on alcohol hasn't deterred you in the slightest (or, you just skipped it altogether) and you are still a regular drinker, let's get you determined to take in more water during your binges. Alcohol is a diuretic. It's not the water in alcohol that makes you pee so frequently; it's the diuretic effect. This is where the water is lost and where the dehydration comes from. The headache in the morning (along with the ridiculous thirst accompanying it) is the clearest indicator of this dehydration.

What's the best way to avoid a hangover? Don't drink.

Or, don't pee. Let me know how that works out...

Yeah, you're not hearing any of that. OK, do this instead—for every alcoholic drink you decide to pound, drink the same quantity of water as a chaser. Do this with every drink you drink during your binge. Will this make it safe and healthy to drink alcohol? No, but it might prevent you from dying from dehydration in the middle of the night.

What about fancy bottled waters, mineral water and sparkling water? There's a lot of controversy about bottled purified waters. Along with the ridiculous price markup and perceived environmental distress, many companies have been caught misrepresenting the purity of their water. So, this is another area for more research. Also, read labels on bottled water. You'd be surprised at what can be added while the manufacturer is still allowed to call the product "water." Some have added sodium, acids, flavorings, sweeteners as well as other additives.

Electrolytes are one of these other potential additives. Some common electrolytes used as additives are:

Sodium
Potassium
Magnesium
Phosphorous
Calcium

In active persons, these are lost when they sweat. For them, electrolyte waters could be of some benefit so long as electrolytes are the only additive in the water. And please don't even think about Gatorade after a workout. Sugar is not a necessary electrolyte.

APPENDIX I: NOW THAT YOU'RE PALEO

Well, you've made it. You have bucked the system, broken all your food addictions and are hanging tough with your own way of eating. It would serve you well at this point to never forget a few things:

1.) *You are in a vast minority*. Lots of people have heard of paleo eating. Many more have tried it out. Not so many have made an unwavering commitment to follow the eating plan as the ultimate authority for living their lives.
2.) You are *viewed as a fanatic* by most people who don't share your zeal for healthful living. You may even have to deal with angry, hostile charges directed at your lifestyle. So be ready.
3.) Be thoughtful and compassionate when sharing your eating habits. The majority of people in the world really still believe deep down that whole grains are ultra-healthy and animal fats are the death knell of humanity. What is undeniable proof of this eating plan's miraculous health benefits for you hasn't been experienced by them.

In this appendix, I am going to share some of the things I've learned in my time doing this that have helped me to stay the course. It has become such an adopted lifestyle for me now that a reversion back to my former ways could honestly never happen. It isn't even the slightest bit tempting.

If you have any bit of doubt remaining in you about the makeup of this eating plan, this is where I will address those lingering concerns. Here are a few areas which might still leave you wondering:

1.) *"Am I eating enough food?"* This is a great question because there should be no comparison of how much food you used to eat with how much you eat now. It should be no contest. If you're not eating less frequently and consuming much less at each sitting than you did when you ate anything you pleased, then there's a problem. If this *really* is the case (it would be rare, but it can happen), you can fix it with fat. This situation could befall someone who makes the switch over to this plan but sticks primarily to eating fruits and vegetables for every meal, forgoing fats such as meats, cheeses, nuts etc. I will talk a lot more about this in the later appendix regarding making this switch and staying vegan, but the key for you would be to force fat into every sitting. If you're making broccoli a meal, for example, make sure it is sautéed in lots of avocado oil or ghee. This will help prevent you from overeating and should keep you from wanting anything else for much longer than naked broccoli would. As far as "getting enough" goes, I am a grown man and I still am quite surprised at the very meager quantity of food that fills me up in a given day since I changed my eating habits. You should only eat if you feel hunger. And there really shouldn't be much of a desire for you to "super-size" things anymore. I typically eat one meal a day. This isn't because I am forcing myself to fast. It is because that is what my body wants. I don't listen to cravings or tradition. I listen strictly to what my body says. I eat at other times of the day but dinner is my only real *meal*. My other feedings usually consist of coffee, a few spoonfuls of almond butter or a couple slices of grass-fed cheese. I treat my morning coffee indulgence as food by loading it with fat in the form of grass-fed, unsalted butter (you heard that right) and coconut oil or full-fat cream and coconut oil. This gets blended into a frothy treat that regularly gets drank more often in the day than just first thing in the morning. So, I suppose it would be "breakfast" if this first feeding of the day had to have a name. But try really hard to get out of the habit of calling your meals by name. That's the conventional way to do it and we're not following convention anymore. Never eat because you think you haven't eaten enough food for the day. That would be silly. Get in tune with, learn to listen to and, most of all, *trust your body* when it comes to what and when you will eat.

2.) *"Am I getting the right ratio of nutrients?"* Since when did you start thinking about this? Not while you were pounding Ding-Dongs and Hot Pockets in the days prior to changing your eating habits, surely. But, I am glad it concerns you now. It wasn't easy to get anything in your system that would have been good for you back then. However, now you could hardly screw it up if you tried. Your approved list of foods is so stocked with nutrients that the selection of anything from it ensures abundant nutritional value. And you also have your body to assist you. If your body needs vitamin C, it never fails that you will start desiring an orange or some broccoli or something else that can provide the nutrient for you. You probably won't notice this. This goes on behind the scenes all the time when your body operates at peak performance while being optimally fueled. It's nothing like a craving.

3.) *"Can I have a cheat day every now and then?"* This seems like a harmless and reasonable idea, doesn't it? If I eat really fantastic for a few weeks with no slip ups, why can't I reward myself with a day of eating anything I want? Well, this is an old-school, low-fat diet way of thinking. Low-fat diets do nothing to cure cravings and food is usually rationed on top of that so the dieter is always starving and wanting more food. Cheat days (which include eating rules going out the window and quantities and types of foods being eaten having no boundaries whatsoever) are almost necessary within these types of diets. But, there is a two-fold problem with combining cheat days with what you are doing now. 1.) You're not dieting so you don't need cheat days. You get to eat whatever you want, whenever you want (as long as you stick to your approved list). This is a great way to live/eat. Why do you need a cheat day? 2.) Cheat days lead to *cheat weeks* and more. And you will be headed down the slope toward the bottom of the ravine again trying to find the point where you will get "back on track." Remember my bowling ball fired out of a cannon analogy? This is a bad place to be. Don't start the ball rolling.

4.) *"I miss pizza."* Yes, I'm sure you do. Now stop, before you do yourself some real harm. In the first section of this book I talked about replacements for your addictions—gluten-free options for gluten and sugar-free ones for sugar. Well those days are behind us now. Forget how the rest of the world eats and quit lamenting what you used to eat (and still think you sorely miss). If you ate pizza now, I bet you'd hate how it makes you feel (but, don't do it in case you really like it and wind up proving me wrong). This is a psychological problem more than anything else. Your brain still has recollection of the cravings that pizza gave you and also remembers the suppression of those cravings that eating pizza would create. This actually tricked you into thinking it tasted even better than it did because it solved your "hunger" like nothing else could. It tickled your brain's pleasure receptors as a result of the drugs hidden within it. That's what you *really* miss. You don't miss pizza. Any kind of replacement pizza you try to make now will always fall short of the outrageous pedestal upon which you have placed gluten-filled, toxic pizza in your mind. So, stop trying to make "pizza." It's not going to measure up. Logically, it will take some time to get over pizza. I understand. But, you should realize that you are fully rehabilitated and you don't need replacements for poisonous foods. The better tactic is to create unique new dishes that you can't live without. By the way, *pizza* here is a metaphor for whatever it is you really might have thought would eventually break you down.

5.) *"My grocery store isn't very paleo-friendly."* I believe you. Mine isn't either. It is why I mostly shop at health food markets. Now, I'm not talking about a store where they sell only vitamin supplements. That would be of no help to you. Health food markets are basically a grocery store with a health food slant. Two of the largest chains that I know of are Sprouts and Whole Foods Market, but there are others. Just understand that you don't have carte blanche to buy whatever you want at these stores. They're still full of a whole lot of crap you can't eat. But, they'll have a lot more of what you can eat. You still have to read labels *very carefully* but you might actually wind up with some processed foods in your cart that meet all the criteria for this eating plan. You won't be able to accomplish that very often at a regular grocery store. These markets also typically have a better selection of grass-fed, uncured, pasture-raised, free range and other meats generally regarded as "healthier." Local farmer's markets will be another great resource for you. Always make sure to read the labels, where provided (or simply ask questions about what it is you're buying).

6.) *"What about foods you don't mention in this book?"* Did I cover everything you are ever going to have a question about with regard to this new eating plan of yours? I highly doubt it. I tried, but I doubt it. Therefore, you are going to have to trust your research skills. You have been honing them all during the process of switching over to this eating style so they should be pretty refined at this point. There are a lot of things you might come across as you start spending more time in the produce section of your grocery store or hanging out more at your local health food market, that might cause some wonder for you. If it's a new food you'd like to try, do this:

a. Determine if it is in a raw state or if it may have been processed. This is a big determinant of how you should approach it. Raw is best. You can always figure out how to prepare it (whatever it is we're talking about here) by searching for recipes online. It is amazing what you'll find help with when it comes to exotic foods (or foods that are exotic to you). If it is processed, get busy scanning the ingredient list. You know how to do this by now.

b. If it is a raw food, plug the item into an internet search in order to ascertain the nutritional data for the item. I found such data for crickets (yes, the bug), so I am sure whatever you find will have some info on it.

c. Search paleo forums and see if anyone is talking about it. There is broad disagreement generally going on in these forums. So it's best to either go with your gut or with the consensus (if you have no feeling about it either way).

d. Determine if it is anti-nutritious. See if it contains such things as lectins, saponins or phytic acid.

e. Make sure it doesn't belong to a food category that you have excluded already such as legumes.

f. Steer clear if it contains enough starch or sugar to cause an insulin response (blood sugar spike).

You don't want your new find to be an energy-sapping, nap-inducer that makes you fat, now do you? It can't be that tasty.

APPENDIX II: CAN I BE PALEO AND VEGAN?

"It's ok to eat fish cause they don't have any feelings." - Kurt Cobain (from the song "Something in The Way" by Nirvana)

Let me start by saying this is a very touchy subject so I will try to tread lightly. My stance is I don't *hate* animals but I feel that for a human diet to be optimal, it needs to include them. This isn't based on opinion or personal ethics. As low fat diets fall out of favor, more is discovered about the actual role and practical necessity of animal fats within the human body. This also covers other nutrients found primarily (or exclusively) in animal products. But, this appendix is not necessarily intended to be a discussion on whether or not eating animal meats is healthy.

I respect all of the reasons why people would adopt a vegan or vegetarian lifestyle. They all have merit and range from ethical and spiritual platforms to a sincere belief that animal products are harmful to human health. You don't hear about too many meat allergies though, so I might not believe you if you try to sell me that as your reasoning.

In case I get a little bit smarmy in my delivery, I probably don't have to worry about too many vegans/vegetarians reading this anyway. This is a paleo book and most of them don't read paleo books because it is pretty universally agreed upon (by paleo advocates and scientists alike) that cavemen ate meat.

The main reason for writing this is not for me to get some jabs in at vegetarians. It is really to illuminate some of the difficulties with the vegan/vegetarian eating style and to discourage you from it at all costs in case you get any crazy ideas. I was one (strict vegetarian) once, for what I thought were health reasons. My biggest problem with adhering to the lifestyle was the same one I encountered while I was trying out low-fat, high-carbohydrate diet plans—not enough fat in the diet to sustain satiety. Although, I didn't know that was the problem at the time. I just knew I didn't feel any healthier whatsoever during my time eating as a vegetarian. And I was always starving. And tofu does not taste like meat.

The foremost difficulty for the vegan/vegetarian is that they need to tirelessly work to make up nutrients. These are elusive nutrients for them that are found in animal products in abundance and in everything else in very scant quantities (or not at all). These are primarily vitamins A, B_6, B_{12}, D, K_2, the minerals *calcium*, *iron* and *zinc* and the macro-nutrient *protein*. There is also a need to make up for a typical lack of *omega-3* essential fatty acids.

The easiest way to address how a reduction (or elimination) of animal products in the diet would align with paleo thinking is to examine vegan/vegetarian divisions one by one. I will list these in order from the most minimally restrictive of animal products to strict elimination:

1.) Flexitarian. This is an odd one to me. It's considered *semi-vegetarianism*. Huh?! Who's the (oxy)moron that came up with that term? Can one be *semi* vegetarian? This basically refers to someone who has consciously determined that they will eat *less* animal meats— a *reducetarian* (I didn't make that up). Honestly, why have a category for this? Pretty much seems like a flexitarian could be anybody, from someone who only eats meat for special holiday occasions to someone like me who doesn't eat meat for breakfast but has it for dinner. This is truly *anybody who isn't vegetarian*. It most definitely is not a category of vegetarianism. I couldn't find any criteria for how a *flexie* (my term) is supposed to measurably reduce their intake. Crazy, man. Crazy. Nice try, though. Since this doesn't qualify as a vegetarian category for me, I won't even attempt to describe how it might work within a paleo-inspired eating format. You flexies can figure that out for yourselves.

2.) Pescatarian (Pescetarian). This group (along with Kurt Cobain) says "it's ok to eat fish." All varieties of fish and all seafood types are generally approved but all other meats are not. Adding fish and seafood at the exclusion of all other meats is not so bad at all from a nutritional standpoint and will almost eliminate the need to search elsewhere for missing nutrients. Vitamin B_{12} content varies greatly amongst fish and seafood varieties. If you're concerned with getting enough B_{12}, you should research this further. Also, increased seafood consumption ups the ante of mercury risk if you worry about that sort of thing.

3.) <u>Porcotarian</u>. Can you guess what this one eats? Pork—ok; other meats—no bueno. I'm not actually sure if it is a real category by itself as I couldn't find much corroboration for it. But it does appear as a combination category as seen in category #5 below. Like pescetarians, this category of vegetarian shouldn't find themselves in much of a nutritional crisis from missing nutrients. Pork seems to have enough of all of the nutrients typically lacking in meatless diets that there isn't much cause for concern here.

4.) <u>Pollotarian</u>. Eats chicken and no other meats. Pretty much the same situation as with the other two semi-vegetarian (*cough*) categories above. Amazing how eliminating meat from the human diet leads to deficiencies in many *critical* nutrient categories while adding any kind of meat whatsoever back into the diet cures this problem instantaneously. Message there? Ah, who knows?

5.) <u>Combination Vegetarian</u>. Any combination of 2 or more of the above 3 categories, such as a *pollo-pescetarian*. A combining of all three results in a *pollo-porco-pescetarian*. Well, I am pretty sure I would never feel pompous enough to trumpet this label describing myself to anyone. I think I would just sheepishly say "I don't eat red meat" instead. But, those in this category should have no problems either; no deficiencies to really worry about.

6.) <u>Lacto vegetarian (Lactarian)</u>. These (along with ovo-vegetarians and lacto-ovo-vegetarians below) are a category that feel that animal slaughter is unconscionable. However, they seem to be alright with *animal slavery*. Animals can provide them with dairy products (lacto vegetarian), eggs (ovo vegetarian) or both (lacto-ovo vegetarian) as long as they don't have to lose their lives for them. Now we will start to see the potential for real deficiencies springing up in the categories from this point forward. Lactarians do need to watch their B_{12} levels. Cottage cheese and yogurt (full-fat versions please) have the highest concentration of this vital nutrient.

7.) <u>Ovo vegetarian (Eggetarian)</u>. Allows eggs only; no meats. Even harder to get enough B_{12} within this category. Eggs also lack sufficient levels of vitamin A, B_6, calcium and iron to really be helpful.

8.) <u>Lacto-ovo vegetarian (Ovo-lacto vegetarian)</u>. Allows eggs and dairy; no meats. Pretty much in the same boat as their lactarian friends.

9.) <u>Vegetarian</u>. The best description for a true vegetarian is one who does not eat any animal products of any kind. They usually eat this way based on strict religious or health beliefs and not on their own moral grounding. Suitable levels for avoiding deficiencies of vitamins B_{12} and K_2 can *only be obtained from animal sources*. Plant sources can provide some (although, often *negligible*) quantities of other missing nutrients. I am not going to go over any of that here. If you decide to forgo eating animal products, you'll need a better guide than this book anyway, believe me.

10.) <u>Vegan</u>. Now, these guys are the ones I truly respect the hell out of. I say, if you're going to do it, go all-in and be one of these. They have adopted a moral stance and they are sold out for it. Really devout vegans go to great lengths to make sure that *everything* that touches their lives must not be traceable in any way to an animal source. On the other hand, the hypocrites in this group (who *incorrectly* call themselves vegan) still wear leather, eat Jell-O and affix things with glue. As much as I love the resolve of a devoted vegan, they really have their work cut out for themselves in getting proper nutrition from the foods they eat. Research this diet vigorously before ever attempting to take it on for yourself. It really can be a dangerous undertaking to become vegan (or one of the stricter varieties of vegetarian).

I really don't understand the adoption of a moral platform for any of these above categories with the one exception of *veganism*. If your reason for subscribing to one of these philosophies is for your own spiritual or health ideals, that is a whole other thing. But, to me, *to object to animal cruelty as a grounds for changing your lifestyle* means the practice will never be tolerable to you in *any form in which it is conceivable*. If you can't buy in on those grounds only (and become devoutly vegan), then I say find something else to stand for. Otherwise, you're a walking contradiction despite your good intentions.

Before concluding this discussion, we should talk about the *quality* of protein that the vegan/vegetarian has available to them. Protein in foods is made up of amino acids. Of these amino acids, some are considered *essential* while others are *non-essential*. The non-essential type (such as alanine, asparagine and glutamic acid, for example) are called as much because the body can manufacture them. They do not need to be culled from dietary sources. The nine essential ones (histidine, isoleucine, leucine, lysine, methionine, phenylalanine, threonine, tryptophan, and valine), on the other hand, must be extracted by the body from food sources. Animal proteins like red meats, chicken, eggs, seafood and dairy products contain all of the essential amino acids. The only plant sources known to be as complete (thus, they are named *complete proteins*) are quinoa and soy. Well, right away there is a problem for you if you are considering becoming a paleo vegan. You don't eat soy. And, quinoa is really not recommended. The grim reality when it comes to such a consideration is you will be starved of some essential amino acids. You will not be getting complete proteins in your diet any longer. You will have to research what the long-term ramifications of that choice would be. However, getting your dietary protein from a variety of sources (plant-based *and* animal-based) ensures you will never face this problem. Therefore, don't experiment with any of the so-called vegetarian options above if you can help it. Flexitarian doesn't count as vegetarian. You can limit animal products all you want (as a flexie would) just don't give them up if you are bent on achieving optimum health.

APPENDIX III: CONVERTING A FAMILY OVER TO PALEO-STYLE EATING

Now here is a legitimate conundrum—converting a family over to this way of eating.

No excuse for deciding *not* to take on the eating style outlined in this book seems more warranted than this one. The argument is typically heard in this way.

"I can switch over to paleo-style eating without a problem, but I wouldn't want to force it on my family."

You wouldn't? Why wouldn't you? You have come to realize that processed food is sheer poison. Is it better that you let your family continue to eat it rather than "force" a new lifestyle on them?

Trust me, they'll get over it. Just like you did.

My family actually thanks me for "forcing" them to eat this way.

"Well, then maybe I will just eat this way so they don't have to be inconvenienced."

Do you have any idea how tired you will soon grow of making two different meals for everyone whenever it's time to eat? Your dedication to this new lifestyle will not last very long, frankly. Since you've decided that they shouldn't suffer, your resolve soon vanishes and you quickly go back to eating like everyone else in the family. The problem is you are too fresh on the scene to not be tempted by all of your former food favorites still being fed to them, while you eat something you aren't so taken with yet. You won't survive this; you will crack. It also is extremely expensive to be buying enough food to prepare separate sittings for everyone.

So, you could always drag them along and not tell them that you're doing it. If you've decided that you are all-in on the plan and not going back, then start them at day one of the 21-day gluten rehabilitation phase and sequence them through the rest of the steps in this book until their approved lists look just like yours. Maybe they won't notice.

A very difficult place to keep children on the right eating path is at school. You can send them with the very best food accompanied by your very best of intentions and they will still find someone who will trade a bag of Cheetos for last night's sautéed broccoli. And you'll never know. But stay the course. Eventually, your kids will come to realize that it's the Cheetos that cause their stomach pains.

Yet, another objection to trying to make an entire family become paleo eaters is the prohibitive cost of healthy food. Now, I will agree that health foods (that comply with this eating plan) seem to cost more than not-so-healthy options. Organic produce usually costs more than other produce. In reality, the word organic, along with grass-fed, pasture-raised, free-range, cage-free, hormone-free and antibiotic-free are all labels that typically are attached to a higher price tag. But, I do not agree that you will be spending more on food than you have been. It is actually more likely that you will spend less once everyone has adapted to eating this way. Assuming you've converted them properly, everyone will eat less at each sitting and all should eat less overall so that you can continue to splurge on the good stuff at your local health food market. Finding proper food to snack on is an initial problem. This is where a lot of the expense can go because these types of foods (i.e., the ones that truly meet the requirements for this eating style) are expensive. But snacking is a habit that can be easily broken once the whole family is adapted to this program. And they won't miss it. That is unless snack time is a regular family ritual at a predetermined time each day (or night). In that case, you have some convincing to do.

APPENDIX IV: THE TIMING OF MEALS AND FASTING

This is an emerging science, so I will tell you what I know of it which will be sprinkled with my own findings from self-experimentation. The concept I will be referring to in this appendix is called *intermittent fasting*.

Intermittent fasting allows certain feeding windows during the day within which the person fasting will permit themselves to eat. Outside of these predetermined time ranges, they do not eat. However, there is no right formula for fasting intermittently and I have seen lots of variations. Here's a relatively common one. A person sets an 8-hour window of time in a day for feeding of 1:00 pm until 9:00 pm. They permit themselves to eat anything inside of this window and nothing else outside of it. This is usually the schedule for eating that they follow for several days or for as long as they decide to fast in this way. A person who fasts intermittently *and* adheres to the eating plan outlined in this book *only eats from their approved list* inside of this window. Other methods for this type of fasting prescribe taking 24 hour periods off from eating. This can be every other day (which is excessive) down to one day of ceased eating in a one-week period. Others delineate different feeding windows such as stopping eating each night by 6:00 pm with no more food eaten until the next morning. But, fasting windows can include a lot of other combinations of starting and stopping times for eating as well.

So why do this? Well, it has shown promise in promoting weight loss. Outside of this reason, though I wouldn't necessarily say it is a great idea.

The general idea of intermittent fasting actually does somewhat echo my urgings to consider feeding yourself outside of the norm of giving meals names and planning meal times. My thought is that the frequency and size of feedings in a day should vary, unique to the day before and based simply on a person's desire to eat (or not). This is especially true of those eating according to the plan laid out in this book who are free from the influence of cravings. So intermittent fasting in the way just described means there is no "breakfast" to be had, nor will there be a meal called "lunch." I really like intermittent fasting for this reason. But it's still very forced and leaves nothing up to your ability to read your own body. I still prefer skipping meals based only on when you feel your body is telling you to do so, but this method of forced fasting can help condition you for exactly that. And you'll probably lose extra weight in the process.

So let me tell you what I learned from fasting intermittently.

1.) Breakfast is overrated. This is a blasphemous statement for most to hear. And, it goes back to more conditioning. Almost anyone can tell you that the reason you get sleepy before lunch is because you're running low on carbs and should have eaten a bigger breakfast. Is this really what we used to think? Please don't tell me you've read this far into this book and still believe it. *"But, breakfast is the most important meal of the day."* I'm not convinced at all that it is. But, regardless, you certainly don't want to screw it up with carbs of any kind. They will positively have you feeling like hell for most of the rest of the day. If you do the 1-9 fast, breakfast is skipped altogether. And the crazy thing is, if you are truly adapted to this eating plan, you will probably also skip lunch and make it well past 1:00 pm rather painlessly. You will drift into ketosis (fat-burning) at your body's first indication of an incoming nutritional shortfall. You will pleasantly burn ketones at a steady rate and never feel sleepy. Instead, you should feel much better throughout the day. However, if you are not yet fully adapted to eating according to the plan of this book, your cravings will convince you that you are going to die before it even gets close to lunch time.

2.) I prefer to *supplement* my fasting with food whenever necessary. This is almost as oxymoronic as the concept of a semi-vegetarian, I know. But, it is how I do it. If my goal for planning a fast is to shed a few pounds, I see no reason why a cup of coffee with healthy fats added to it is going to spoil things. My definition of fasting simply means *not eating meals*. It would be no different than a juice fast, which seems to be all the rage these days (except juice of any kind is horrible for you so don't consider doing this for any reason; it is only being mentioned for illustration purposes). A little fat ensures I don't feel inclined to make a meal for myself before the end of whatever time range I set for myself to fast. A tablespoon of cashew butter is food but it certainly isn't a meal. Intermittent fasting is far more successful (for me, anyway) when the option exists to supplement with tiny servings of fat (and *only* fat) in this way. It all depends on your definition of fasting I guess and how strict you want to get with it. But, I pretty much exist in a constant cycle of this type of fasting (because I only really ever eat one regular meal a day—in the evening) so I have plenty of experience with it. My biggest finding is that total starvation seems counter-productive to the efficiency that simply eliminating whole meals can have in the process of losing weight utilizing fasting. You are far more likely to cave in and ruin any effect that supplemented fasting might have had if you set your fasting range too broad and allow yourself no option for supplementing with fat if you feel the need. This supplementation should *only happen if you are feeling uncomfortable during the fast*. It should not be planned out (just like your normal eating days shouldn't have planned meals and meal times). In fact, it would always be best to ride out the entire fast period you've set for yourself without taking in any food to ensure you stay in ketosis for as long as possible. But, knowing the option to supplement with fat exists guarantees I will make it; even if my target for fasting is a 24-hour period or longer. I never short myself of water while fasting. In reality, water sometimes does a great job of curbing your feelings of hunger as well. Try it first, before resorting to fat to do the job.

3.) Intermittent fasting really works. It exists outside the paleo community and is regularly prescribed for weight loss to many without including a recommendation to modify one's diet at all. If it can work under those circumstances, imagine what it can do for you and your approved foods list. It's not that you're necessarily eating less food while fasting intermittently, it's that you are guaranteeing periods of ketosis which wouldn't probably otherwise happen if you constantly fed yourself throughout the day. Once you arrive at ketosis, your body settles in for the ride and can get pretty comfortable doing so. Really, the biggest enemy of ketosis and the one that spoils it sooner than any other factor is your brain. It is best to be really distracted with activities when attempting to fast. The more opportunities you have during the fast to "think" about what you're doing (and especially, how long it's been since you ate anything), the harder it will be to stay strong.

My suggestion, if you decide you'd like to try intermittent fasting, is to start by just skipping a meal in the morning (notice I didn't call it "breakfast"). So, for ease of understanding, let's just say no food until 11:00 am. Then adjust the duration of your fast from there. Don't feel bad about still having coffee (loaded with fat), if that's your ritual. I would never take away your coffee as I wouldn't wish that kind of cruelty on my own worst enemy. If your coffee doesn't have fat in it, it may have an opposite effect than what you're going for. The caffeine could actually *stimulate* hunger in the absence of fat to counter the effect and then you really will have a long way to go until your fast period is supposed to end.

Experiment with different ways of fasting. Try new eating windows and different durations. The smaller the feeding window, the more time spent fasting. You usually will be in a state of ketosis while sleeping so make sure to factor periods of sleep into the fasting side of the equation. Lots of intermittent fasting enthusiasts rave about 24 hour and longer fasts. You will have to try longer fasts out on your own, if you're interested. I find them really annoying and unnecessary as I can achieve great results with much smaller fasting windows.

APPENDIX V: THE AUTHOR'S PERSONAL APPROVED LIST—A TEMPLATE FOR CREATING YOUR OWN

This appendix is designed to show you what a written approved list might look like. It is built from all of the lists laid out in previous chapters that were intended to get you going with creating your final approved list. It shows all of the items from those lists and then includes strikethroughs for the items I am not so fond of, have never tried or which don't agree with me personally. Don't let these strikethroughs deter you from trying things on this list. For example, I have organ meats stricken from this list, but I am trying to develop a taste for them because they are so incredibly nutrient dense. I have decided to list everything under the heading of <u>green</u> or <u>yellow</u>. These are meant to model two of the colors in a traffic signal—*green for go* (eat without reservation) and *yellow for caution* (can lead to allergenic/other reactivity, insulin response or is inhibiting to weight loss).

<u>Fruits (Green)</u>:
Avocado
Cucumber
Pumpkin
Squash (Acorn, Banana, Buttercup, Butternut, Summer)
Yellow Squash
Zucchini Squash

<u>Vegetables (Green)</u>:
Artichoke
Asparagus
Belgian Endive
~~Bok Choy~~
Broccoflower
Broccoli
Brussels Sprouts

Cabbage (green and red, Napa or Chinese, Savoy)
Carrots
Cauliflower
Celery
Coconuts
Endive
~~Escarole~~
~~Fennel~~
Garlic
Green Onions
Greens (Turnip, Beet, Collard, Mustard)
~~Jerusalem Artichoke~~
Kale
Kohlrabi
~~Leeks~~
Lettuce (Boston, Iceberg, Leaf, Romaine)
Mushrooms
~~Okra~~
Onion (green, red, Spanish, yellow, white)
Radicchio
Radishes
~~Rhubarb~~
Shallots
Spinach
Sprouts (seed sprouts only; no legumes)
~~Swiss Chard~~
Turnip
Water Chestnuts
Watercress
Yucca/Cassava

Poultry and Avian Game Meats (Green):
Chicken
Cornish Hen/Cornish Game Hen
~~Duck~~
~~Goose~~
~~Guineafowl~~
~~Pheasant~~
~~Quail~~

~~Squab~~
Turkey
~~Wild Turkey~~

Fresh Pork Cuts (Green):
Back Ribs
Belly
Blade Steak
Boneless Loin/Loin Roast
Chops (Shoulder, Sirloin, Boneless, Loin Chop, Rib Chop)
Country-Style Ribs
Crown Roast
Ground Pork
Rib Roast/Rack Of Pork
Shoulder/Boston Butt
Spareribs
Tenderloin

Fresh Red Meat Cuts—these can be beef, bison/buffalo, elk or game varieties (Green):
Back Ribs
Brisket
Chuck Roast
Filet Mignon
Flank Steak
Flat Iron
Ground Meat
~~Organ Meats/Offal~~
Rib Roast
Ribeye Steak
Sirloin Steak
Skirt Steak
Strip Steak
T-Bone Steak
Tenderloin Roast
Top Round Roast
Tri-Tip Roast

Nuts and Seeds (Yellow):

Almonds
Brazil Nuts
Cashews
Chestnuts
~~Filberts (or, Hazelnuts)~~
~~Hickory Nuts~~
~~Litchi~~
Macadamia Nuts
Pecans
Pine Nuts
Pistachios
Poppy Seeds
Pumpkin Seeds
Sesame Seeds
Sunflower Seeds
Walnuts

Fruits (Yellow):
Apple
Apricot
Asian Pear
Banana
~~Bitter Melon~~
Blackberries
Blueberries
~~Boysenberries~~
~~Cantaloupe~~
~~Casaba Melon~~
Cherries
Dates (ripe, soft; not dried)
~~Figs (not dried)~~
~~Gooseberries~~
Grapefruit
Grapes
~~Honeydew Melon~~
~~Horned Melon~~
Kiwifruit
~~Kumquat~~
Lemons

Limes
~~Loquat~~
~~Lychee~~
Mandarin Oranges
Mangos
~~Mulberries~~
Nectarines
Oranges
Papayas
Passion Fruit
Peaches
Pears
~~Persimmons~~
Pineapple
Plantains
Plums
~~Pomegranate~~
~~Prickly Pear (Cactus Pear)~~
~~Pummelo (Chinese Grapefruit)~~
~~Quince~~
Raspberries
Strawberries
Tangelo
Tangerines
Watermelon

Vegetables (Yellow):
Beets
Jicama
Parsnip
~~Rutabaga~~
Sweet Potato
Yams

Nightshades (Yellow):
Bell Peppers (green, red, orange, yellow)
Eggplant
Goji Berries

Hot Peppers (cayenne, jalapeno, habanero, serrano, chili peppers, paprika)
Pimentos
Potatoes (red, white, yellow, Yukon Gold, Russet)
Tomatillos
Tomatoes

Dairy Products (Yellow):
Cream
Half and Half
Milk

Fermented Dairy Products (Yellow):
Cheeses
Kefir
Sour Cream
Yogurt

Lacto-Fermented Foods (Yellow):
Cheese
Cucumber
~~Kimchi~~
~~Sauerkraut~~
Vegetables
Yogurt

Mixed Ferments—yeast, bacteria or other (Yellow):
Kefir
Kombucha
~~Water Kefir~~

Mold Fermented Foods (Yellow):
Bleu Cheese
Brie Cheese
Camembert Cheese
Gorgonzola Cheese
Roquefort Cheese
Stilton Cheese

Fish and Seafood (Yellow):
~~Abalone~~
~~Amberjack~~
~~Anchovy~~
Atlantic Cod
Atlantic Salmon
Basa/Swai
Bass
Black Sea Bass
Catfish
Chilean Sea Bass
~~Clams~~
~~Cockle~~
Crab (King, Dungeness, Snow)
Crawfish/Crayfish
Flounder
Grouper
Haddock
Halibut
Lobster (~~Spiny~~, Norway, Rock)
Mackerel
Mahi-Mahi
Monkfish
Mullet
~~Mussels~~
~~Ocean Perch~~
~~Octopus~~
~~Oysters~~
Pacific Cod
Pike
Pollock
Rockfish
Salmon (~~Chinook~~, King, Sockeye, Alaskan, Pink, ~~Coho~~)
~~Sardines~~
Scallops
Sea Bass (European)
~~Sea Urchin~~
~~Shad~~
Shark

Shrimp/Prawns
~~Smelt~~
Snapper
Sole
~~Squid (Calamari)~~
Sturgeon
~~Sunfish~~
Tilapia
Trout
Tuna
~~Whiting~~

Preserved Pork Products (Yellow):
Bacon
Canadian Bacon
Capicola
Coppa
Culatello
Ham
~~Hot Dogs/Frankfurters~~
Mortadella
Pancetta
Pepperoni
Porchetta
Prosciutto
Salami/Salame/Salumi (Hard, Genoa, Soppressata, Peppered, Cotto)
Sausages (Bratwurst, Italian, Breakfast, ~~Chorizo~~, Andouille)
Summer Sausage/Kielbasa

Preserved Red Meats (Yellow):
Beef/Game Sausages or Hot Dogs
~~Canned Meats~~
Corned Beef
Jerky/~~Processed and Formed Meat Snacks~~/Dried Meats
Luncheon Meats

CPSIA information can be obtained
at www.ICGtesting.com
Printed in the USA
LVHW010012040119
602730LV00007B/206

9 781530 098101